PSYCHIATRIC MEDICINE

The Psychiatrist's Guide
to the Treatment of
Common
Medical Illnesses

MAHENDRA J. DAVE, MD
Distinguished Fellow of the
American Psychiatric Association
Past President of the Medical Staff at
Georgia Regional Hospital
Department of Psychiatry
Morehouse School of Medicine
Atlanta, Georgia

KURT P. MICELI, MD
Department of Internal and Psychiatric Medicine
University of Virginia
Charlottesville, Virginia

POONAM MODHA, MD
Department of Psychiatry and Human Behavior
Brown University Medical School
Providence, Rhode Island

Wolters Kluwer | Lippincott Williams & Wilkins
Health
Philadelphia · Baltimore · New York · London
Buenos Aires · Hong Kong · Sydney · Tokyo

Acquisitions Editor: Charles W. Mitchell
Managing Editor: Sirkka Howes Bertling
Marketing Manager: Kimberly Schonberger
Project Manager: Bridgett Dougherty
Manufacturing Manager: Kathleen Brown
Design Coordinator: Risa Clow
Production Services: Laserwords Private Limited, Chennai, India

Library of Congress Cataloging-in-Publication Data

Dave, Mahendra J.
  Psychiatric medicine : the psychiatrist's guide to the treatment of common medical illnesses / Mahendra J. Dave, Kurt P. Miceli, Poonam Modha.
    p. ; cm.
  Includes bibliographical references and index.
  ISBN 978-0-7817-8408-5
  1. Clinical medicine. 2. Psychotherapy patients—Medical care. 3. Psychiatrists.
I. Miceli, Kurt P. II. Modha, Poonam. III. Title.
  [DNLM: 1. Therapeutics. 2. Diagnosis. 3. Psychiatry—methods. WB 300 D246p 2008]
  RC48.D25 2008
  616.89'18—dc22

                                                              2007035915

PSYCHIATRIC MEDICINE

The Psychiatrist's Guide to the Treatment of
Common
Medical Illnesses

PREFACE

We, as psychiatrists, are often called upon to treat patients with common medical illnesses. As an intern, resident, or an on-call doctor on a psychiatry service, you may be the only physician available, particularly on evenings, nights, and weekends to treat these common medical illnesses. As we grow in experience as psychiatrists, our knowledge on the treatments of the medical illnesses may lag behind. We have experienced the above dilemma, and have wished for a helpful guide.

This concise book is intended to fill that need.

As a practical guide, this book provides the basic understanding and significance of the commonly ordered laboratory studies (Part I), information on common medical illnesses and their specific treatments (Part II), and information on certain syndromes in psychiatry, some of which are potentially lethal, which require prompt medical attention (Part III).

Although this book was written with the psychiatrist in mind, we believe that it will also be useful to our colleagues from other medical specialties where the illnesses discussed in this guide are not encountered on a daily basis.

Mahendra J. Dave, MD
Kurt P. Miceli, MD
Poonam Modha, MD

CONTENTS

PART 2 ▪ CLINICAL MEDICINE

PART 3 ■ SOME IMPORTANT PSYCHIATRIC SYNDROMES

PSYCHIATRIC MEDICINE

The Psychiatrist's Guide
to the Treatment of
Common
Medical Illnesses

Part 1

Laboratory Medicine

Laboratory test results are accompanied by the normal reference range for the laboratory where the tests are performed. These may differ slightly from laboratory to laboratory.

The normal value is that which is achieved by 95% of the normal population, or one that falls within two standard deviations from the mean for that test.

URINALYSIS

Glucose	Negative
Bilirubin	Negative
Ketones	Negative
Specific gravity	1.001 to 1.035
Hemoglobin	Negative
pH	4.8 to 8.0
Total protein	Negative
Nitrite	Negative
Leukocyte esterase	Negative
Urobilinogen	0.1 to 1 Ehrlich unit per dL

a. Glucose

Positive in diabetes mellitus, other endocrine conditions (hyperthyroidism, Cushing's syndrome), other pancreatic conditions (pancreatitis, carcinoma), renal conditions (renal tubular dysfunction), central nervous system (CNS) conditions (meningitis, cerebrovascular accidents), pheochromocytoma, severe burns, infections, and fractures.

b. Bilirubin

> **NOTE:**
>
> The bilirubin found in urine is the conjugated form, as the unconjugated form is not soluble.

Positive test results occur in jaundice secondary to liver disease and obstructive biliary tract disease.

c. Ketones

Positive in starvation, diabetes mellitus

d. Specific gravity

Decreased:
    Overhydration
    Diabetes insipidus
    Decreased concentrating ability of the kidneys
Increased:
    Dehydration
    Fever

    Increased fluid loss—vomiting, diarrhea
    Diabetes mellitus

e. Hemoglobin

Positive in renal disease, renal calculi, skeletal muscle or cardiac muscle injury, extreme excercise, urinary tract infection

f. pH

Decreased:
    Metabolic/respiratory acidosis
Increased:
    Urinary tract infection, with urea splitting bacteria
    Hypokalemic, hypochloremic acidosis—urine is paradoxically alkaline

g. Total protein

Positive in renal dysfunction, multiple myeloma, fever, severe stress, leukemia, pre-eclampsia

h. Nitrite

> **NOTE:**
>
> Most, but not all, bacteria in urine reduce urine nitrate to nitrite.

Positive nitrite indicates presence of bacterial infection.

i. Leukocyte esterase

> **NOTE:**
>
> White blood cells release esterase.

Positive test indirectly establishes pyuria.

j. Urobilinogen

> **NOTE:**
>
> Conjugated bilirubin in the intestinal tract gets converted to urobilinogen by bacterial action. Fifty percent of the urobilinogen is reabsorbed, and is recirculated through the liver, and a small amount is excreted in urine.

Decreased:
    Obstructive liver disease
Increased:
    Hemolytic jaundice
    Cirrhosis

Hepatitis
Infectious mononucleosis
Urinalysis—microscopic

WBC 0 to 2	Normal
RBC 0 to 2	Normal
WBC >5	Infection
WBC 5 to 50	Chronic infection
WBC >50	Acute infection
Nitrite+	Infection
Epithelial cells+	Infection

Urinalysis—Culture and Sensitivity Reports

REMEMBER:

Urinalysis that reports <100,000 colony-forming units of a specific pathogen in an asymptomatic patient does not require treatment. However, a symptomatic patient, or one who has urological problems or has undergone a urinary tract procedure, requires a much lower colony count threshold for treatment. (See Chapter 2.57.)

NOTE:

Urinalysis that reports >100,000 colony-forming units, but of multiple organisms with no predominant pathogen is generally consistent with a contaminated specimen.

The report on the sensitivity of the organism to the medications is reported as numbers which follow letters I, R, or S, where

I stands for Intermediate,

R stands for Resistant, and

S stands for Susceptible.

The report shows the minimum inhibitory concentration that produced destruction of the organism.

For example, the report may read:

Amoxicillin/clavulanic acid	$I = 16$
Ampicillin	$R \geq 16$
Cefoxitin	$S \leq 4$
Gentamicin	$S \leq 32$
Nitrofurantoin	$R \geq 160$

For the medications that the organism is resistant to, the higher the number, the more the resistance.

For the medications that the organism is susceptible to, the lower the number, the more susceptible the organism is to the effect of the medication.

COMPLETE BLOOD COUNT

WHITE BLOOD CELL COUNT

African American adults 3,200 to 10,000 per mm^3; other adults 4,500 to 10,500 per mm^3 (panic value: <1,500/ mm^3); elderly male 4,200 to 16,000 per mm^3; elderly female 3,100 to 10,000 per mm^3

WHITE BLOOD CELLS—DIFFERENTIAL COUNT

Neutrophils 2,500 to 7,000 per mm^3: adult 50% to 70%; elderly 45% to 75%

Lymphocytes 1,500 to 4,000 per mm^3: adult 25% to 40%

NOTE:

Lymphocytes consist of B lymphocytes and T lymphocytes. B lymphocytes control the antigen B antibody reaction. T lymphocytes are the master immune cells, and are further differentiated into helper T cells (CD4), killer cells, cytotoxic cells, and suppressor T cells (CD8).

Eosinophils 100 to 300 per mm^3: adult 1% to 3%

Basophils 40 to 100 per mm^3: adult 0.5%to 1.0%; elderly average 1%

Monocytes 200 to 600 per mm^3: adult 4% to 6%; elderly average 10%

RED BLOOD CELL COUNT

Adult male 4.5 to 6.0 million per mm^3; adult female 4.0 to 5.0 million per mm^3; elderly male 3.7 to 6.0 million per mm^3; elderly female 4.0 to 5.0 million per mm^3

HEMOGLOBIN

Adult male 13.5 to 18.0 g per dL; adult female 12.0 to 16.0 g per dL; elderly male 11.0 to 17.0 g per dL; elderly female 11.5 to 16.0 g per dL

HEMATOCRIT

Adult male 40% to 54%; adult female 36% to 41%; elderly male 38% to 42%; elderly female 38% to 41%

MEAN CORPUSCULAR VOLUME

Adult 80 to 98 μm^3; elderly male 74 to 110 μm^3; elderly female 78 to 100 μm^3

MEAN CORPUSCULAR HEMOGLOBIN

Adult 27 to 31 pg; elderly male 24 to 33 pg; elderly female 23 to 34 pg

MEAN CORPUSCULAR HEMOGLOBIN CONCENTRATION

Adult 32% to 36%; elderly male 28% to 36%; elderly female 30% to 36%

RED CELL DISTRIBUTION WIDTH

11.5 to 14.5 Coulter S

PLATELET COUNT

150,000 to 400,000 per mm^3

MEAN PLATELET VOLUME (MPV)

7.4 to 10.4 μm^3

a. Neutrophils

Increased:

> Acute infections—bacterial, viral (first few days), fungal, rickettsial, and so on
>
> Inflammation or tissue damage—myocardial infarction, burns, crush injury, acute appendicitis, acute cholecystitis, acute pancreatitis, dermatitis, thyroiditis and collagen diseases, such as rheumatoid arthritis, gout, systemic lupus erythematosus
>
> Acquired hemolytic anemia
>
> Medications—corticosteroids, lithium, digitalis, epinephrine
>
> Hematologic—acute hemorrhage
>
> Myelocytic leukemia
>
> Idiopathic or familial

Decreased:

> Infections—typhoid, acquired immunodeficiency syndrome (AIDS), other viral diseases, overwhelming infections particularly in the elderly
>
> Lymphocytic leukemia, monocytic leukemia
>
> Iron deficiency, folic acid deficiency, and aplastic anemias
>
> Systemic lupus erythematosus, rheumatoid arthritis, cirrhosis
>
> Medications—many antibiotics, tranquilizers

b. Lymphocytes

Increased:

> Chronic bacterial infections—tuberculosis, pertussis, brucellosis
>
> Acute viral infections—hepatitis, infectious mononucleosis, mumps, acute human immunodeficiency virus (HIV) infection, and so on
>
> Acute lymphocytic leukemia, chronic lymphocytic leukemia, Hodgkin's disease, multiple myeloma
>
> Endocrine dysfunction—adrenocortical hypofunction, thyrotoxicosis

Decreased:

> Collagen vascular diseases—systemic lupus erythematosus

Aplastic anemia, bone marrow aplasia
Adrenocortical hyperfunction—Cushing's syndrome, and so on
Oral corticosteroids
Sarcoidosis, renal failure

c. CD4 count

> **NOTE:**
>
> CD4 count is the number of absolute lymphocytes that are stained with CD4.

Increased:
Diurnal variation—morning values are approximately half the peak evening values
Decreased (CD4 count <200 cells/μL or a lymphocyte percentage below 14%):
AIDS

> **REMEMBER:**
>
> Depressed CD4 count is a reliable indicator of imminent opportunistic infection.

d. Eosinophils

Increased:
Allergic conditions—asthma, allergic reaction to medications, allergic rhinitis, atopic dermatitis
Parasitic and fungal disorders—scabies, coccidioidomycosis, mucocutaneous candidiasis (thrush)
Collagen vascular diseases—rheumatoid arthritis, periarteritis nodosa
Malignancy—eosinophilic leukemia, Hodgkin's disease, malignant lymphoma, and malignancy of bone, brain, ovary, testes
Pulmonary eosinophilic syndromes—tropical eosinophilia
Decreased:
Adrenocortical hyperfunction—Cushing's syndrome, and so on
Oral corticosteroids
Acute infections, burns, shock, inflammation

e. Basophils

Increased:
Basophilic leukemia, Hodgkin's disease
During the healing stage of infections and inflammations
Acquired hemolytic anemia
Decreased:
Adrenocortical hyperfunction—Cushing's syndrome, and so on
Oral corticosteroids, epinephrine
Acute infections, burns, shock, inflammation

f. Monocytes

Increased:
    Monocytic leukemia
    Malignancies of bone, brain, bladder, liver, gastrointestinal cancers, and so on
    Recovery from acute bacterial infections
    Recovery from inflammatory conditions
    Sickle cell and hemolytic anemias
    Collagen vascular diseases—systemic lupus erythematosus, rheumatoid arthritis
    Sarcoidosis, ulcerative colitis
    Chronic high dose corticosteroids
Decreased:
    Aplastic anemia
    Use of corticosteroids

g. Red blood cell count (RBC), hemoglobin (Hb), hematocrit (Hct)

Decreased:
    Anemias
Elevated:
    Polycythemia vera

h. Mean corpuscular volume (MCV)

Decreased:
    Iron deficiency anemia
    Thalassemia
    Sickle cell anemia
    Hemolytic anemia
    Sideroblastic anemia (hereditary, lead poisoning, pyridoxine deficiency)
    Hereditary spherocytosis
Increased:
    Folic acid or vitamin B_{12} deficiency anemia
    Pernicious anemia
    Reticulocytosis
    Liver disease

i. Mean corpuscular hemoglobin (MCH), mean corpuscular hemoglobin concentration (MCHC)

Decreased:
    Iron deficiency anemia
    Sideroblastic anemia
Increased:
    Hereditary spherocytosis

j. Red cell distribution width (RDW)

> **NOTE:**
>
> RDW measures the difference in width of the RBCs.

RDW is an early manifestation of most anemias, including deficiency anemias (iron, folate, B_{12}), hemolytic anemias, and acquired sideroblastic anemias from lead poisoning and pyridoxine deficiency, which impair enzymes involved in the formation of heme.

RDW differentiates two forms of microcytic anemias—Iron deficiency anemia has a high RDW whereas thalassemia has a low RDW.

k. Platelet count

Increased:
　　Polycythemia vera
　　Chronic myelocytic leukemia
　　Collagen vascular disease
　　Anemias—iron deficiency anemia, and hemolytic anemia following splenectomy
　　Metastatic carcinoma
　　After trauma, hemorrhage, surgery, splenectomy

Decreased:
　　Ineffective manufacture of platelets may occur in chronic alcoholism, megaloblastic anemias, aplastic anemia, congenital thrombocytopenias
　　Purpura—idiopathic thrombocytopenic purpura, thrombotic thrombocytopenic purpura, anphylactoid purpura
　　Lupus erythematosus, chronic lymphocytic leukemia, disseminated intravascular coagulopathy
　　Hypersplenism secondary to cirrhosis, myelofibrosis with myeloid metaplasia, leukemias, lymphomas

l. Mean platelet volume (MPV)

Increased:
　　Purpura—idiopathic thrombocytopenic purpura
　　Myeloproliferative disease—leukemia, myeloid metaplasia, polycythemia vera
　　Megaloblastic anemia
　　Splenectomy
　　Massive hemorrhage

Decreased:
　　Wiscott-Aldrich syndrome

BASIC CHEMISTRY PANEL

Sodium	135 to 145 mmol per L (panic value: <125 or >155 mmol/L)
Potassium	3.5 to 5.0 mmol per L (panic value: <3.0 or >6.0 mmol/L)
Chloride	101 to 112 mmol per L
CO_2	22 to 32 mmol per L (panic value: <15 or >40 mmol/L)
Anion gap	3 to 11 mmol per L
Glucose, fasting	60 to 100 mg per dL (panic value: <40 or >500)
Blood urea nitrogen (BUN)	8 to 20 mg per dL
Creatinine	0.5 to 1.5 mg per dL
BUN/creatinine ratio	10:1 to 20:1
Calcium	8.5 to 10.5 mg per dL (panic value <6.5 or >13.5 mg/dL)
Aspartate aminotransferase (AST)	10 to 40 IU per L
Serum osmolality (calculated)	275 to 300 mOsm per kg H_2O (panic value <240 or >320 mOsm/kg H_2O)

a. Sodium 135 to 145 mmol per L (panic value: <125 or >155 mmol/L)

REMEMBER:

Patients may remain asymptomatic if a severe hyponatremia (110 mEq/L) is gradual, whereas an acute decrease to a level of 125 mEq per L may be symptomatic, and will require intravenous saline replacement.

Hyponatremia may cause increased pulse, hypotension, lethargy, muscle weakness, headaches, anxiety, muscle twitches. Acute hyponatremia may present with altered mental status, and seizures. Hypernatremia may accompany increased pulse, weakness, signs of dehydration, such as dry tongue, thirst, restlessness, confusion, neuromuscular excitability, seizures, coma.

Increased:
  Excessive sodium intake, dehydration, severe vomiting, and severe diarrhea
  Cushing's syndrome (excess of cortisol)
  Aldosteronism
  Nephrogenic diabetes insipidus
  Medications—methyldopa, reserpine, and so on

Decreased:

Syndrome of inappropriate antidiuretic hormone secretion (SIADH)

Polyuria, vomiting, diarrhea, perspiration, burns

Hypoaldosteronism (adrenal insufficiency)

Dilutional hyponatremia can occur with hyperglycemia due to shift of water from intracellular to extracellular space. Edema secondary to congestive heart failure (CHF), cirrhosis, or nephrotic syndrome will show hypervolemic hyponatremia.

Renal insufficiency, renal tubular acidosis

Medications—carbamazepine and diuretics, such as furosemide (Lasix), thiazides

b. Potassium 3.5 to 5.0 mmol per L (panic value : <3.0 or >6.0 mmol/L)

REMEMBER:

Cardiac arrest can occur with potassium levels above 7.0 mmol per L or below 2.5 mmol per L.

Clinically, hypokalemia can cause decreased pulse, increased respiration, cardiac arrhythmias, fatigue, myalgia, muscle weakness, leg cramps, nausea, vomiting, diarrhea, dizziness, irritability, confusion, and mental depression.

Hyperkalemia causes decreased pulse, weakness, abdominal cramps, numbness or tingling in the extremities, oliguria or anuria.

A decrease in plasma potassium of 1 mEq per L represents a total body potassium deficit of 200 to 400 mEq.

Increased:

Hemolyzed serum

Renal insufficiency—acute or chronic, with oliguria

Adrenocortical insufficiency (acute, chronic—Addison's disease)

Crush injuries, muscle necrosis, burns

Diabetic ketoacidosis

Medications—spironolactone, triamterene, and so on

Decreased:

Aldosteronism, Cushing's syndrome

Vomiting, diarrhea, malabsorption syndromes

Diuretic and laxative abuse, surreptitious vomiting (as in eating disorders)

Familial periodic hypokalemic paralysis

Dehydration, starvation, excessive perspiration

Renal tubular acidosis

Diabetic acidosis

Medications/foods—adrenocorticosteroids, chlorothiazide, thiazide diuretics, furosemide, ethacrynic acid, excessive licorice, excessive glucose, and so on

c. Chloride 101 to 112 mmol per L

Increased:

Hyperparathyroidism

Hyperchloremic metabolic acidosis

Renal disease—glomerulonephritis, renal tubular acidosis, pyelonephritis, polycystic renal disease

Severe dehydration

Medications—ammonium chloride, cortisone

Decreased:

Vomiting, diarrhea, nasogastric suction, excessive sweating, burns

Emphysema gives rise to chronic respiratory acidosis.

Metabolic alkalosis

Diabetic acidosis

SIADH

Addison's disease

Cushing's syndrome (adrenocortical hyperfunction) from cancer

Medications—loop diuretics

d. CO_2 22 to 32 mmol per L (panic value: <15 or >40 mmol/L)

> **NOTE:**
>
> The carbon dioxide content approximates the amount of bicarbonate in serum.

Increased:

Metabolic alkalosis

Chronic respiratory acidosis with compensation

Decreased:

Metabolic acidosis

Chronic respiratory alkalosis with compensation

When vacutainer tubes are underfilled

e. Anion gap 3 to 11 mmol per L

> **NOTE:**
>
> Anion gap is the difference between the cations (positive ions) Na and K, and the anions (negative ions) chloride and bicarbonate, that is, CO_2.

Increased:

Renal failure

Ketoacidosis (uncontrolled diabetes mellitus, starvation, anorexia nervosa, alcoholic)

Lactic acidosis

Poisoning from salicylates (Aspirin), methanol, antifreeze (ethylene glycol), paraldehyde, paint thinner

Decreased:

Multiple myeloma, hypermagnesemia, hyponatremia, hypoalbuminemia (nephrosis, glomerulonephritis)

f. Glucose, Fasting 60 to 100 mg per dL (panic value: <40 or >500)

Increased:

Diabetes mellitus, prediabetes, adrenocortical hyperfunction (Cushing syndrome, cortical excess), hyperpituitarism (acromegaly), hyperthyroidism, cancer of pancreas

Decreased:

Adrenocortical hypofunction, hypopituitarism, hyperinsulinism, cirrhosis, alcoholism

g. BUN 8 to 20 mg per dL

Increased:

Renal insufficiency (nephritis, renal failure)

Prerenal causes (from decreased renal blood flow)—congestive heart failure, shock, adrenal insufficiency

Postrenal causes—urinary tract obstruction, renal vein thrombosis, dehydration, gastrointestinal bleeding

Decreased:

Malnutrition, hepatic failure, overhydration, SIADH

h. Creatinine 0.5 to 1.5 mg per dL

NOTE:

Creatinine is produced from the breakdown of creatine in skeletal muscle.

Increased:

Renal insufficiency (acute or chronic), and muscle necrosis

Decreased levels are of no known clinical significance

i. BUN/creatinine ratio 10:1 to 20:1

Increased ratio:

Occurs in dehydration, as BUN increases with dehydration, but creatinine does not.

Decreased ratio:

Secondary to prerenal causes, from decreased renal blood flow—congestive heart failure, shock, adrenal insufficiency

Secondary to postrenal causes, from urinary tract obstruction, renal vein thrombosis

---

REMEMBER:

The ratio remains unchanged in renal disease as there is a proportionate increase in BUN and creatinine.

---

j. Calcium 8.5 to 10.5 mg per dL (panic value <6.5 or >13.5 mg/dL)

Increased:

Hyperparathyroidism

Cancer of bone, breast, bladder, lungs, cervix, prostrate, kidneys, multiple myeloma

Drug induced—vitamins A and D, calcium, thiazides, estrogen

Decreased:

> Hypoparathyroidism, pseudohypoparathyroidism, malabsorption syndromes, vitamin D deficiency, renal failure, magnesium deficiency, pancreatitis with necrosis

k. Asparate aminotransferase (AST) (Serum Glutamic-oxaloacetic transaminase[SGOT]) 10 to 40 IU per L

NOTE:

Tissue distribution of AST is widespread.

Increased:

> Liver diseases
>
> Heart—acute myocardial infarction, acute myocarditis, congestive heart failure
>
> Skeletal muscle disease—muscular dystrophy, dermatomyositis
>
> Red blood cell—severe hemolytic anemia, megaloblastic anemia
>
> Other—acute pulmonary infarction, acute renal failure, acute pancreatitis, infectious mononucleosis, third degree burns, and so on.
>
> Medications—heparin therapy, oral contraceptives, salicylate, acetaminophen, carbamazepine, and so on

Decreased:

> B_6 (pyridoxine) deficiency, chronic dialysis, pregnancy

l. Serum osmolality (calculated) 275 to 300 mOsm per kg H_2O (panic value <240 or >320 mOsm/kg H_2O)

NOTE:

Serum osmolality is a sensitive indicator of the number of dissolved particles in the serum, such as creatinine, electrolytes, glucose, proteins, and urea.

Increased:

> Dehydration, diabetes insipidus, and conditions in which there is an increase in BUN, glucose, sodium.

Decreased:

> SIADH, overhydration, and sodium loss

LIVER PROFILE

Bilirubin, total	0.1 to 1.2 mg per dL
Alkaline phosphatase	41 to 133 U per L
Aspartate aminotransferase (AST)/serum glutamic-oxaloacetic transaminase (SGOT)	10 to 40 U per L (laboratory specific)
Alanine aminotransferase (ALT)/serum glutamic-pyruvic transaminase (SGPT)	7 to 56 U per L (laboratory specific)
Lactate dehydrogenase (LDH)	88 to 230 U per L (laboratory specific)
Albumin	3.4 to 4.7 g per dL

a. Bilirubin, total 0.1 to 1.2 mg per dL

NOTE:

Bilirubin is produced by catabolism of heme, which results from hemoglobin of old red blood cells, from bone marrow normoblasts, and from cytochrome and myoglobin. It circulates in plasma as unconjugated bilirubin (also called *indirect bilirubin*), which is the insoluble form, and is bound to albumin. The hepatocytes in the liver conjugate bilirubin with glucuronic acid to form water-soluble conjugated bilirubin (also called *direct bilirubin*).

When the laboratory reports one level of bilirubin, it is the total bilirubin.

Increased:
   Hepatitis
   Liver damage
   Obstructive liver disease
   Hemolysis
   Sickle cell anemia
   Fasting
   Malnutrition
   Reaction to medications

b. Alkaline Phosphatase 41 to 133 U per L

Increased:
   Hepatic conditions—hepatitis (viral, toxic, alcoholic), cirrhosis, infectious mononucleosis, carcinoma head of pancreas, cholestasis

secondary to intrahepatic and extrahepatic causes, congestive heart failure

Bone conditions—fractures, malignancy, hyperparathyroidism, rickets

Other—leukemia, ulcerative colitis, reparative phase of myocardial and pulmonary infarction. Ectopic production of alkaline phosphatase occurs in malignancy of cervix, ovary, lungs, breast, and colon.

Decreased:
  Hypothyroidism
  Hypophosphatasia
  Pernicious anemia
  Zinc and magnesium deficiency

c. AST/SGOT 10 per 40 U per L (laboratory specific)

NOTE:
Tissue distribution of AST is widespread.

Increased:
  Liver diseases
  Heart—acute myocardial infarction, acute myocarditis, congestive heart failure
  Skeletal muscle disease—muscular dystrophy, dermatomyocytis
  Red blood cell—severe hemolytic anemia, megaloblastic anemia
  Other—acute pulmonary infarction, acute renal failure, acute pancreatitis, Infectious mononucleosis, third-degree burns and so on.
  Medications—heparin therapy, oral contraceptives, salicylate, acetaminophen, carbamazepine and so on
Decreased:
  B$_6$ (pyridoxine) deficiency
  Chronic dialysis
  Pregnancy

d. ALT/SGPT 7 to 56 U per L (laboratory specific)

NOTE:
Tissue distribution—liver, kidneys

Increased:
  Liver diseases
  Acute renal infarction
  Heart—congestive heart failure, acute myocardial infarction
  Skeletal muscle disease
  Heparin therapy
  Acute pancreatitis

e. LDH 88 to 230 U per L (laboratory specific)

> **NOTE:**
>
> Tissue distribution of LDH is widespread.
> Five types of LDH isoenzyme have been identified.
> LDH-1 and LDH-2 predominate in heart, red blood cells and kidneys.
> LDH-3 predominates in lungs.
> LDH-4 and LDH 5 predominate in liver and skeletal muscles.

Increased:
  Liver disease
  Heart—congestive heart failure, acute myocardial infarction
  Lungs—pulmonary infarction, active pulmonary disease
  Brain—cerebrovascular accidents
  Skeletal muscle disease
  Trauma, tissue necrosis, shock
  Blood—megaloblastic anemia, hemolysis, transfusions, heparin
    therapy

f. Albumin 3.4 to 4.7 g per dL

Increased:
  Dehydration
Decreased:
  Hepatic insufficiency
  Nephrosis
  Glomerulonephritis
  Neoplasms
  Chronic infections
  Malnutrition

1.5

THYROID PANEL

Thyroid-stimulating hormone (TSH)	0.35 to 5.5 μIU per mL
Thyroxine (T_4)	4.5 to 12.0 μg per dL (100 mL)
3,5,3'-Triiodothyronine (T_3) uptake	24% to 39%
Free thyroxine index (FTI)	1.5 to 4.5

a. TSH 0.35 to 5.5 μIU per mL

Increased:
  Primary hypothyroidism
  Thyroiditis
  Cirrhosis of the liver
Decreased:
  Anterior pituitary gland dysfunction
  Hypothalamic dysfunction
  Klinefelter's syndrome

b. T_4 4.5 to 12.0 μg per dL (100 mL)

> **NOTE:**
>
> T_4 gives the value of tetraiodothyronine that is in the free unbound form and the protein-bound form. The latter is primarily bound to thyroxine-binding globulins, and prealbumin.

Increased:
  Primary and secondary hyperthyroidism
  Increased thyroxine-binding proteins (pregnancy, acute hepatitis)
Decreased:
  Primary and secondary hypothyroidism
  Decreased thyroxine-binding proteins (malnutrition, nephrosis)

c. T_3 uptake 24% to 39%

> **NOTE:**
>
> T_3 resin uptake test is an indirect measurement that reflects the percent of binding sites occupied on the thyroxine binding globulin

Increased:
  Hyperthyroidism
  Conditions with decreased thyroid-binding globulin such as malnutrition, nephrotic syndrome
Decreased:
  Hypothyroidism
  Conditions with increased levels of thyroid-binding globulin, such as pregnancy, acute hepatitis

d. FTI, T_7 1.5 to 4.5

> **NOTE:**
>
> This test is a mathematical measurement of T_4 multiplied by T_3 resin uptake. This corrects for the abnormalities of thyroxine binding.

Increased:
  Hyperthyroidism
Decreased:
  Hypothyroidism

TESTS FOR SYPHILIS

Rapid plasma reagin (RPR) and Venereal Disease Research Laboratory test (VDRL) for syphilis can be false positive, and so fluorescent treponemal antibody absorption test (FTA-ABS) is done to confirm the diagnosis of syphilis.

REMEMBER:

Titers of RPR, VDRL or FTA-ABS may remain positive after treatment in patients who have higher initial titers, or who had a more advanced disease, or who have had repeated infections.

A stable RPR titer of 1:2 to 1:8 in an individual who has been treated in the past requires no treatment. Treatment is required if the current titer is at least three times more as compared to a past post-treatment titer.

LABORATORY TESTS FOR MYOCARDIAL INFARCTION

Troponin-I (cTnI)	<0.05 ng per mL
Creatine kinase MB (CKMB)	<16 units per L or <4% of total CK
Lactate dehydrogenase (LDH)	88 to 230 units per L (laboratory specific)
Aspartate aminotransferase (AST, SGOT)	10 to 40 units per L (laboratory specific)

NOTE:

Tests for troponin and CKMB are relatively specific for acute myocardial infarction (MI), and have replaced the tests for cardiac isoform of LDH, and AST.

> **REMEMBER:**
>
> Laboratory tests for cardiac enzymes can often make a more accurate diagnosis of an acute MI as 20% of acute MIs are silent, and the specific electrocardiogram (EKG) findings are often not present in 50% of the patients.

a. Treponin-I (cTnI) <0.05 ng per mL

> **NOTE:**
>
> Troponins are proteins that regulate the actin-myosin interaction of the heart muscle. Tests have been developed to measure tropnonin T (which binds to tropomyosin) and troponin I (which inhibits the interaction of actin with myosin).

The levels of troponins begin to rise in the blood 3 to 4 hours after an acute MI, and remain detectable for 10 to 14 days.

b. CKMB <16 units per L or <4% of total CK

> **NOTE:**
>
> The isoenzyme MB of CK (CPK) is relatively specific for the cardiac muscle, although it can be increased after pulmonary embolism, severe muscle injury, or vigorous exercise.

CKMB begins to enter the blood 4 to 8 hours after the acute MI, the level peaks in approximately 24 hours, and returns to normal within the next 2 to 3 days.

c. LDH 88 to 230 units per L (laboratory specific)

> **NOTE:**
>
> In MI there is an LDH flip (when LDH-1 level becomes >LDH-2 level).

Level rises 12 to 24 hours after the infarction, peaks in 2 to 5 days, and returns to normal over the next 7 to 10 days.

d. AST, SGOT 10 to 40 units per L (laboratory specific)
Levels peak in 2 to 3 days, and return to normal in 5 to 7 days.

TESTS FOR DIABETES MELLITUS AND PREDIABETES

According to American Diabetic Association (ADA) position statement, 1994, the diagnosis of diabetes is made if

1. A patient has the symptoms of diabetes (polyuria, polydipsia, and unexplained weight loss) and has a casual plasma glucose level (i.e., a random plasma glucose level, irrespective of time of the last meal) of $\geq$200 mg per dL.
   OR
2. Fasting plasma glucose (FPG) (i.e., the patient has had no caloric intake for at least 8 hours) of $\geq$126 mg per dL.
   OR
3. Oral glucose tolerance test (OGTT) which shows a plasma glucose level of $\geq$200 mg per dL, at 2 hours after an oral load of 75 g of anhydrous glucose dissolved in water.
   AND
   A repeat confirmation of any of the above three criteria on a separate day.

   Impaired fasting glucose (IFG) is FPG of 100 to 125 mg per dL
   Impaired OGTT is 2-hour postload plasma glucose level of 140 to 199 mg per dL
   Patients who have IFG and/or impaired glucose tolerance are considered to have prediabetes, which is a risk factor for diabetes.

ADA recommends that, for adequate glycemic control, the patients with DM have the following:

1. Glycated (glycosylated) hemoglobin (Hg A_{Ic}) of <7.0%
2. Preprandial plasma glucose of 90 to 130 mg per dL
3. Postprandial plasma glucose of <180 mg per dL.

a. Hemoglobin A_{Ic}

   Glycated (glycosylated) hemoglobin (Hg A_{Ic}) 3.9% to 6.9% (method dependent)

NOTE:

Hemoglobin A makes up 97% of normal hemoglobin. Approximately 4% to 6% of this gets glycated (glycosylated) by a nearly irreversible, nonenzymatic action when hemoglobin gets bound to glucose. This is Hg A_{Ic}. The other glycohemoglobins are formed by phosphorylation of glucose or fructose with hemoglobin, to form Hg A_{Ia} and Hg A_{Ib}.

> **REMEMBER:**
>
> The glycated hemoglobin reflects the average blood glucose level over the preceding 2 to 3 months. Use Hg A_{1C} level to make therapeutic decisions regarding medication adjustments.
>   It is not recommended for the diagnoses of diabetes.

Increased:
    Poorly controlled diabetes
    Iron-deficiency anemia
    Spleenectomy
    False positive in thalassemia
Decreased:
    Chronic blood loss
    Hemolytic anemia
    Pregnancy
    Chronic renal failure

1.9

TESTS FOR MONITORING ANTICOAGULANT THERAPY

Prothrombin time (PT) 11 to 15 seconds (panic value: $\geq$30 seconds)

> **NOTE:**
>
> Thromboplastin converts prothrombin (factor II) to thrombin. The strength of the thromboplastin used in the PT determination varies with the manufacturer, which can then give different prothrombin time results. This difference is therefore standardized by use of the international normalized ratio (INR).

PT-INR for patients on stable oral anticoagulant therapy is 2.0 to 3.0 for patients being treated for deep vein thrombosis, and is 3.0 to 4.0 for patients with mechanical heart valves.
Partial thromboplastin time (PTT) 60 to 70 seconds.
Activated partial thromboplastin time (APTT) 25 to 35 seconds.

a. PT 11 to 15 seconds (panic value: $\geq$30 seconds)

NOTE:

Prothrombin time is the most sensitive assay used to monitor the efficacy of oral anticoagulants, such as warfarin (brand Coumadin), bishydroxy-coumarin (dicoumarol), and anisindione (Miradon). PT is relatively insensitive to the effect of heparin.

REMEMBER:

The PT is maintained at 1.3 to 1.5 times the control in seconds for effective therapy of deep vein thrombosis, and is maintained at 1.5 to 2 times the control in seconds for effective therapy of patients with mechanical heart valves.

Increased:
>   Deficiencies of factors II, V, VII, and X
>   Afibrinogenemia
>   Vitamin K deficiency
>   Liver disease
>   Therapy with oral anticoagulants

b. PTT 60 to 70 seconds.

Activated partial thromboplastin time (APTT) 25 to 35 seconds.

REMEMBER:

PTT and APTT are used to monitor heparin therapy, to monitor replacement therapy in hemophilia, and in detecting disorders of clotting factors and platelets.
>   APTT is more sensitive than PTT.

For effective heparin therapy, the PTT and APTT are maintained at 1.5 to 2.5 times the control values in seconds obtained before heparin therapy.

APTT of more than 100 seconds is associated with spontaneous bleeding.

ANEMIAS

Ferritin: adult male 16 to 300 ng per mL; adult female 4 to 161 ng per mL
Iron   50 to 175 μg per dL
Total iron binding capacity   250 to 460 μg per dL
Transferrin   190 to 375 mg per dL
Vitamin B$_{12}$ (cyanocobalamin)   100 to 700 pg per mL
Folic acid (folate)   3 to 16 ng per mL

a. Ferritin: adult male 16 to 300 ng per mL; adult female 4 to 161 ng per mL

> **NOTE:**
>
> Ferritin is an iron storage protein. Serum ferritin levels reflect the amount of iron stored in the body.

Increased:
   Acute or chronic liver disease
   Hemolytic anemias, megaloblastic anemias, thalassemia
   Inflammatory diseases
   Iron overload (oral or parenteral, hemochromatosis, hemosiderosis)
   Leukemia, Hodgkin's disease, breast carcinoma
Decreased:
   Iron deficiency anemia

b. Iron 50 to 175 μg per dL

Increased:
   Iron overload
   Hemolytic anemias (pernicious anemia, thalassemia)
   Acute hepatitis, alcoholic cirrhosis
Decreased:
   Iron deficiency anemia
   Anemia of chronic disease
   Chronic blood loss
   Chronic renal failure

c. Total iron binding capacity 250 to 460 μg per dL

Increased:
   Iron deficiency anemia
   Pregnancy during the third trimester
   Hemorrhage

Decreased:
- Hemolytic, pernicious, and sickle cell anemia
- Anemia of chronic disease
- Protein deficiency—malnutrition, burns
- Renal failure
- Alcoholic cirrhosis

d. Transferrin 190 to 375 mg per dL

> **NOTE:**
>
> Transferrin is a glycoprotein responsible for transporting iron (from food, or from RBC breakdown product) to the bone marrow for hemoglobin synthesis.

Increased:
- Severe iron deficiency

Decreased:
- Anemias of chronic disease
- Hepatic damage
- Hereditary atransferrinemia
- Iron overload

e. Vitamin B_{12} (cyanocobalamin) 100 to 700 pg per mL

Increased:
- Liver disease—cirrhosis, acute or chronic hepatitis
- Myelocytic leukemia
- Increased dietary intake

Decreased:
- Pernicious anemia
- Malabsorption syndromes
- Pregnancy
- Insufficient dietary intake
- Posterolateral sclerosis

f. Folic acid (folate) 3 to 16 ng per mL

Increased:
- Pernicious anemia
- Vitamin B_{12} deficiency
- Increased dietary intake

Decreased:
- Megaloblastic anemia
- Insufficient dietary intake, malabsorption syndrome
- Alcohol
- Pregnancy
- Liver disease
- Oral contraceptives, phenytoin, primidone, antimalarial medications

PULSE OXIMETRY

The normal reference range for arterial oxygen saturation (Sao_2) is 95% to 100%.

Pulse oximetry measures the oxygen saturation noninvasively, without the need to get the arterial blood gas study. Pulse oximetry is indicated during the emergency management of airway, and to monitor the adequacy of oxygen delivery. Oxygen is generally indicated in patients with acute myocardial infarction, upper airway obstruction, aspiration, sepsis, and in other critically ill patients, including possibly patients with delirium.

> **REMEMBER:**
>
> Oxygen delivery should not be delayed until reading can be obtained on the oximeter.

The pulse oximeter has a clip with a sensor, which is attached to a clean finger over the nail, and a computer screen, which shows the oxygen saturation.

Sao_2 <95% indicates hypoxia, and need for oxygen by nasal cannula.

OTHER MISCELLANEOUS TESTS IMPORTANT TO THE PSYCHIATRIST

a. Magnesium 1.8 to 3.0 mg per dL (panic value: <0.5 or >4.5 mg/dL)

> **REMEMBER:**
>
> In the presence of magnesium deficiency, hypocalcaemia and hypokalemia cannot be corrected without magnesium therapy.

Increased:

Renal insufficiency (acute or chronic), adrenal insufficiency, severe dehydration

Decreased:

Alcoholism (acute or chronic), malnutrition, nephritis, malabsorption syndromes, severe diarrhea, hypocalcaemia, diabetes mellitus

Furosemide, ethcrynic acid, thiazides, calcium, and so on

b. Creatine kinase (CK, CPK) (32 to 267 units, dependent on the method used)

NOTE:

CK has three isoenzymes.
    Fraction 1, isoenzyme BB, present in brain
    Fraction 2, isoenzyme MB, present in heart
    Fraction 3, isoenzyme MM, present in skeletal muscle.

Increase of CK:

Skeletal muscle disease—muscular dystrophies, trauma, polymyositis, severe muscle exertion, and in marathon runners

Heart—acute myocardial infarction, CO poisoning, acute myocarditis

Brain—cerebrovascular accidents, head injury

Part 2

Clinical Medicine

ACETAMINOPHEN (APAP/TYLENOL) OVERDOSE

I. Main pathways for acetaminophen (APAP) metabolism in the normal individual:
   a. APAP (~90%) + glucuronide OR sulfate through conjugation → nontoxic metabolites
   b. APAP (~5%) → toxic NAPQI (N-acetyl-p-benzoquinoneimine), through cytochrome P450... then, rather rapidly... toxic NAPQI + GSH (glutathione) → nontoxic metabolites

---

KEY POINT:

In APAP overdose, the conjugation pathways are overwhelmed, and more APAP goes through P-450, thereby increasing toxic NAPQI. Furthermore, any agent that induces the P-450 system (e.g., ethanol) or decreases GSH increases the risk for APAP hepatotoxicity.

II. Evaluation
   a. Toxic dose = 150 mg per kg or 15 g in a 100-kg adult.
   b. Chronic ingestion of >4 g per day may also be toxic.
III. Diagnostic phases of APAP overdose
   a. First phase (initial 24 hours)—nonspecific findings (gastrointestinal [GI] symptoms, anorexia, pallor, lethargy); Liver function tests (LFTs) start to increase
   b. Second phase (24–72 hours)—clinical (right upper quadrant [RUQ] pain) and laboratory (↑ prothrombin time [PT], ↑ bilirubin, ↑ creatinine) signs of hepatotoxicity
   c. Third phase (72–96 hours)—fulminant hepatic failure (alanine aminotransferase [ALT] and aspartate aminotransferase [AST] >10 K, ↑ PT, ↑ bilirubin producing jaundice)
   d. Fourth phase (4 days–2 weeks)—resolution of liver function and complete recovery (if patient survives)

REMEMBER:

Even those who have taken dangerous amounts of APAP may appear clinically normal and have normal vital signs.

IV. Treatment
   a. Give activated charcoal if patient presents within 4 hours of overdose.

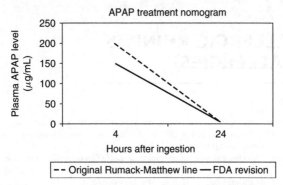

FIGURE 2.1.1 Acetaminophen (APAP) treatment nomogram. FDA, U.S. Food and Drug Administration. (Adapted from Rumack BH, Matthew H. Acetaminophen Poisoning and Toxicity. Pediatrics. 1975;55(6):871–876.)

    i. Ipecac is contraindicated because it produces vomiting which may inhibit PO treatment.

  b. Get APAP level (ideally 4 hours after ingestion to plot on Rumack-Matthew treatment nomogram as shown in Figure 2.1.1).

    i. Those who are above the toxic line should get *N*-acetylcysteine (NAC = Mucomyst).

      1. NAC is equally effective when given between 0 to 8 hours postoverdose.

    ii. If APAP is undetectable and ↑ AST and ALT, then assume patient is in second phase and give NAC.

  c. Get chemistry (blood urea nitrogen [BUN], creatinine), LFTs, PT/partial thromboplastin time (PTT), and monitor at least every day throughout course.

V. NAC therapy

  a. NAC is a precursor of GSH; therefore, GSH synthesis increases and more NAPQI can be made nontoxic.

  b. NAC is best given <8 hours after overdose, but is effective no matter how late the therapy starts.

  c. Dosing

    i. Twenty-hour protocol with IV NAC (U.S. Food and Drug Administration [FDA] approved in 2004)

      1. Loading dose of 150 mg per kg over 15 minutes

      2. Then, 50 mg per kg of NAC infused over 4 hours

      3. Then, 100 mg per kg of NAC infused over 16 hours

    ii. A 72-hour protocol of PO NAC (standard treatment in the United States pre-2004)

      1. Loading dose of 140 mg per kg

      2. Maintenance dose of 70 mg per kg q4h × 17 doses

ALLERGIC RHINITIS (ALLERGIES)

I. Evaluation
   a. Description—inflammatory condition of the nasal mucosa
   b. Clinical—pruritus (severe itching), sneezing, rhinorrhea, and nasal congestion
   c. Mechanism—immunoglobulin E (IgE)-associated response to allergens
   d. Epidemiology—15% to 20% prevalence
   e. Classification
      i. Traditional—seasonal (cyclic pollens) or perennial (year-round allergens)
      ii. New—intermittent (≤ 4 days/week or ≤ 4 weeks) or persistent (> 4 days/week and > 4 weeks).
II. Differential diagnosis for allergic rhinitis
   a. Nonallergic rhinitis
      i. Mechanical/structural (e.g., nasal tumors, foreign body, etc.)
      ii. Infectious
      iii. Vasomotor or idiopathic (e.g., cold air-induced, pressure-induced, odors, etc.)
      iv. Reflex-induced (e.g., postural, gustatory—after ingestion of food, chemical, etc.)
   b. Drug-induced rhinitis
      i. Oral contraceptive pills (OCPs)
      ii. Nonsteroidal anti-inflammatory drugs (NSAIDs) and Aspirin
      iii. Hydralazine
      iv. β-Blockers
   c. Hormonally-induced rhinitis
      i. Pregnancy or menstrual cycle
      ii. Hypothyroidism
      iii. Exercise
   d. Granulomatous rhinitis
      i. Sarcoidosis
      ii. Wegener's granulomatosis
   e. Cerebrospinal rhinorrhea (clear cerebrospinal fluid [CSF] rhinorrhea)
III. Treatment
   a. Intranasal corticosteroid (single most effective class of medications for allergic rhinitis)
      i. Fluticasone (Flonase) 50 μg per spray—administer two sprays per nostril daily.

    ii. Budesonide (Rhinocort) 32 μg per spray—administer one spray per nostril daily.
- b. H$_1$ antihistamines (remember, histamine is the major mediator of allergic inflammation)
  - i. First generation—sedating (drowsy, decreased cognition, motor impairment)
    1. Diphenhydramine (Benadryl) 25 to 50 mg PO TID p.r.n.
    2. Hydroxyzine (Atarax) 25 to 50 mg PO TID p.r.n. or qhs.
  - ii. Second generation (effectiveness much better established than for first generation)
    1. Loratadine (Claritin) 10 mg PO daily
    2. Desloratadine (Clarinex) 5 mg PO daily
    3. Cetirizine (Zyrtec) 5 to 10 mg PO daily
    4. Fexofenadine (Allegra) 120 to 180 mg PO daily (least potential for sedation)
- c. Decongestants—vasoconstrictors affecting α-receptors only helps nasal congestion
  - i. Topical or PO
    1. Pseudoephedrine (Sudafed) 30 to 60 mg q6hrs p.r.n. ($\times$1 week maximum)
- d. Leukotriene receptor blockade (do not appear more effective than antihistamines)
  - i. Montelukast (Singulair) 10 mg PO daily.
- e. Cromolyn (inhibits degranulation of mast cells)
  - i. Cromolyn nasal (NasalCrom) 5.2 mg per spray—administer one spray per nostril TID to QID

2.3

ANAPHYLAXIS

I. Evaluation
- a. Description—acute, potentially life-threatening hypersensitivity reaction with systemic effects
- b. Clinical:
  - i. Cardiovascular—lightheaded and syncope secondary to hypotension
  - ii. Respiratory—rhinitis, sneezing → stridor, chest tightness, shortness of breath, wheeze, respiratory arrest
  - iii. Skin—pruritus, flushing, hives, angioedema
  - iv. Neurologic—anxiety
  - v. Gastrointestinal (GI)—nausea, vomiting, diarrhea, cramping

c. Mechanism—antigen/antibody-mediated response involving immunoglobulin E (IgE)

REMEMBER:

Non–IgE-mediated response that activates mast cells is termed *anaphylactoid.*

---

d. Epidemiology
   i. A total of 500 to 1,000 deaths occur annually in the United States.
   ii. More than 500,000 serious allergic reactions to medications occur annually in hospitals.
e. Risk factors
   i. Age—children have more food-related anaphylaxis; adults more so with antibiotics, stings.
      1. Common foods—peanuts, nuts, fish, shellfish, milk, eggs, sesame
      2. Common drugs—penicillin, sulfa, nonsteroidal anti-inflammatory drugs (NSAIDs), muscle relaxants, contrast, and so on
   ii. Sex—men have a higher occurrence with stings; women with latex, Aspirin, contrast.
   iii. Exposure—the more time since last exposure, the less likely a reaction will transpire.
   iv. Location—occurrence is higher in rural patients than in urban.

II. Management
a. Stop the agent causing the insult.
b. Assess airway, breathing, circulation (ABCs).
c. Treat!

III. Pharmacologic treatment
a. Epinephrine is the drug of choice for immediate therapy during anaphylaxis.
   i. Epinephrine 0.3 to 0.5 mL of a 1:1,000 dilution IM q10min until improvement.
   ii. Note—Glucagon 5 to 15 μg per minute IV may be needed for patients on β-blockers.

REMEMBER:

Volume replacement is essential because anaphylaxis produces an increase in vascular permeability, effectively producing intravascular volume depletion.

---

b. H$_1$ antihistamines—effective in controlling skin symptoms.
   i. Diphenhydramine (Benadryl) 25 to 50 mg q4h to q6h IV/IM p.r.n.

   c. H_2 antihistamines (combination of H_1 and H_2 antihistamines superior to either alone)

      i. Ranitidine (Zantac) 50 mg IV q8h p.r.n. OR 150 mg PO daily p.r.n.

   d. Inhaled β_2-agonist—useful when bronchospasm is present.

      i. Albuterol inhaler 2 puffs q4h p.r.n. OR nebulizer q4h p.r.n.

   e. Corticosteroids—help prevent or decrease late-phase reactions, hence not first-line treatment.

      i. Methylprednisolone (Solu-Medrol) 100 to 250 mg IV q8h p.r.n.

IV. Prevention

   a. First step—find the inciting agent. Avoid it, as well as substances with potential for cross-reactivity.

   b. Prescribe and instruct the patient in using a self-injectable epinephrine (EpiPen).

      i. Write for two EpiPens—one at home and one with the patient at all times.

2.4

ANEMIA

I. Evaluation

   a. Description—a specific decrease in the number of circulating erythrocytes (red blood cells [RBCs]), hemoglobin, and hematocrit

   b. Clinical

      i. If anemia has developed rapidly—hypotension is secondary to loss of blood volume.

      ii. Tissue and organ hypoxia (fatigue, shortness of breath, ± pica, etc.) are seen in either chronic or acute anemia.

      iii. Pallor, hypotension, tachycardia are seen on physical examination.

      iv. Mild anemia in a young, healthy patient may not be noticed until hemoglobin <8 g per dL.

   c. Epidemiology

      i. ♀: 30 of 1,000 of all ages

      ii. ♂: 6 of 1,000 for younger than 45 years; 18.5 of 1,000 for older than 75 years

   d. Diagnostic algorithm

      i. First, look at hemoglobin

	Anemia if Hemoglobin...	
	♀	♂
12–18 yr	<12	<13
>18 yr	<12	<13.5

ii. Second, look at reticulocyte count
  1. If elevated, consider
    a. Hemolysis
      i. Acquired
        1. Immune hemolysis (autoimmune, drug-induced)
        2. Traumatic. Examples include:
          a. Thrombotic thrombocytopenic purpura (TTP)
          b. Disseminated intravascular coagulation (DIC)
          c. Prosthetic heart valves
        3. Hypersplenism
        4. Infection (eg., malaria, clostridia toxin)
        5. Osmotic damage (eg., fresh water drowning)
      ii. Inherited/congenital (eg., G6PD deficiency, thalassemias, hemoglobin S, etc.)
    b. Blood loss (can be acute or chronic)
  2. If not elevated, then check mean corpuscular volume (MCV):
    a. Low MCV
      i. Iron deficiency
      ii. Anemia of chronic disease (some cases)
      iii. Lead poisoning
    b. Normal MCV
      i. Iron deficiency (mild–moderate)
      ii. Anemia of chronic disease (most cases)
      iii. Renal insufficiency
      iv. Bone marrow aplasia/hypoplasia
    c. Elevated MCV
      i. Vitamin B$_{12}$ deficiency
      ii. Folate deficiency
      iii. Hypothyroidism
      iv. Liver disease (eg., alcoholism)
e. Specific considerations
  i. Iron deficiency anemia
    1. Epidemiology—most common cause of anemia worldwide
    2. Clinical—glossitis, koilonychia (nails are flattened; concavities present)

3. Laboratory findings—↓ iron, ↓ ferritin (iron stores), ↑ transferrin (iron delivery protein)
4. Etiology
   a. Blood loss (menstruation; gastrointestinal (GI) bleed from ulcer, malignancy, or hemorrhoids)
   b. Ineffective iron intake. Examples include the following:
      i. Acid reduction treatment—proton pump inhibitors (PPI) and H_2-blockers
      ii. Poor compliance
   c. Not absorbing iron (Celiac sprue, Crohn's disease, pernicious anemia, gastric surgery)
5. Management—investigate blood loss, especially in those older than 50 years, to rule out malignancy
6. Treatment—ferrous sulfate 325 mg PO TID.
   a. Hemoglobin levels should show improvement within 1 to 2 months of therapy.
   b. Side effects (common) include nausea, constipation, diarrhea, abdominal pain.

ii. Vitamin B_{12} deficiency
   1. General—body stores of B_{12} adequate for up to 5 years
   2. Clinical—glossitis, numbness, paresthesias, ataxia, decreased vibratory/position sense
   3. Laboratory findings—↓ B_{12}, ↑ lactate dehydrogenase (LDH), ↑ bilirubin, hypersegmented polymorphonuclear neutrophils (polys)
   4. Etiology—usually the result of the prolonged failure of the body to absorb B_{12}
      a. Most frequent causes—pernicious anemia, Crohn's disease, and so on
      b. Malnutrition (alcoholics, vegetarians)
   5. Treatment—vitamin B_{12} 1,000 μg IM × 5 days, then weekly × 4 weeks, then monthly

iii. Folate deficiency
   1. General—body stores of folate adequate for 2 to 3 months; found in green leafy vegetables
   2. Clinical—glossitis, fetal neural tube defects
   3. Laboratory findings—↓ folate, ↑ LDH, ↑ bilirubin, hypersegmented polymorphonuclear neutrophils (polys)
   4. Etiology
      a. GI absorption difficulties (e.g., Celiac sprue)
      b. Malnutrition (alcoholism, elderly)
      c. Drug therapy with folate antagonists
         i. For example, Methotrexate (MTX), Trimethoprim (TMP)
      d. Increased requirements (pregnancy, dialysis)
   5. Treatment—folic acid 1 mg PO daily.

    f. Psychiatric pearls, pointers, and parallels
        i. Symptom parallels:
            1. Shortness of breath and tachycardia may be mistaken for
                a primary anxiety disorder.
            2. Angina can be a result of anemia and can cause severe
                anxiety.
            3. Fatigue associated with anemia can appear to be a symp-
                tom of depression.
                a. Other neurovegetative symptoms can be present as
                    well.
            4. Pica can be a symptom of anemia and may be mistaken
                for psychopathology.
            5. Symptom of restless legs may be associated with vitamin
                B_{12} deficiency.
        ii. Chronic alcohol use can cause myelosuppression, leading to
            anemia, leukopenia, and thrombocytopenia.

2.5

ANGINA

I. Evaluation
    a. Description—chest pain in conjunction with myocardial
        ischemia, not myocardial necrosis
    b. Types
        i. Typical (all three are present) versus atypical (two are
            present) versus noncardiac (one present)
            1. Pain located in chest, shoulder, arm, or jaw
            2. Worsens with stress (physical or emotional)
            3. Relieved by nitroglycerin
II. Differential diagnosis of acute chest pain
    a. Cardiovascular
        i. Stable angina
        ii. Acute coronary syndrome (ACS)—need hospital admission
            and cardiology care
            1. Unstable angina—myocardial ischemic pain at rest, of
                new onset, or increase in severity
            2. Non–ST elevation myocardial infarction (NSTEMI)
                a. Evidence of myocardial infarction (MI) (+ troponin),
                    but no ST elevation on electrocardiogram (EKG)

3. ST elevation myocardial infarction (STEMI)
   a. Evidence of myocardial infarction (MI) (+ troponin)
   b. Equal to or greater than 1 mm of new ST segment elevation in more than two leads

iii. Aortic dissection—acute sharp chest pain that radiates to the back

iv. Pericarditis/myocarditis—sharp, pleuritic pain that is positional

  b. Non-cardiovascular
     i. Pulmonary (eg., pulmonary embolism—pleuritic chest pain, dyspnea, cough, hemoptysis)
     ii. Gastrointestinal (eg., gastroesophageal reflux disease (GERD), heartburn, etc.)
     iii. Musculoskeletal (eg., costochondritis—this pain may be reproducible on examination)
     iv. Psychiatric (eg., anxiety, etc.)

III. Management of stable angina
  a. Order
     i. EKG—get within 5 minutes of the patient presenting with symptoms suggestive of angina.
        1. Q waves in concordant leads suggest prior infarct.
        2. EKG signs are suggestive of ACS.
           a. ST-segment elevation or depression
           b. Inverted T waves, including "pseudonormalization" of previously flipped T waves
     ii. Stress testing—it is used to risk-stratify patients with angina.
        1. May also use stress testing to diagnose coronary disease as a cause of chest pain
  b. Pathophysiology—patients with angina experience chest pain when O_2 demand is greater than O_2 supply.
  c. Treatment—aims to reverse the pathophysiological imbalance described in the preceding text.
     i. Improve long-term outcomes
        1. Aspirin 81 to 325 mg PO daily
           a. Decreases adverse cardiovascular events by 33% in patients with stable angina.
        2. Clopidogrel (Plavix) 75 mg PO daily—alternate for those who cannot take aspirin
        3. Lipid-lowering agents (eg., statins, etc.)
     ii. Improve symptoms
        1. Nitrates—arterial and venous vasodilators → increase coronary blood flow.
           a. Short-acting
              i. Nitroglycerin 0.3 to 0.6 mg SL q5min p.r.n. (maximum: 3 doses in 24 hours)
           b. Long-acting
              i. Isosorbide mononitrate 30 to 240 mg PO daily

        ii. Nitroglycerin transdermal 0.2 to 0.4 mg per hour patch daily[a]

        iii. Nitroglycerin topical 0.5 to 2 inches topical q4h to q6h[a]

    c. Avoid using with sildenafil (Viagra) due to potential for hypotension → death.

  2. Calcium channel blockers (CCB)

    a. General

      i. Vasodilate coronaries, ↓ peripheral vascular resistance (PVR) and contractility

      ii. Can be used for Prinzmetal's angina (vasospastic angina)

    b. Negative inotropes— (avoid in patients with left ventricle dysfunction)

      i. Verapamil 80 to 160 mg PO TID

      ii. Diltiazem (Cardizem) 30 to 90 mg PO QID

      iii. Nifedipine (Procardia) 10 to 20 mg PO TID

    c. Less negative inotropes— (ok in patients with left ventricle dysfunction)

      i. Amlodipine (Norvasc) 2.5 to 10 mg PO daily

      ii. Felodipine (Plendil) 2.5 to 10 mg PO daily

iii. Improve long-term outcomes and symptoms

  1. β-blockers

    a. General

      i. Goal—lower resting heart rate to 55 to 60 bpm and achieve blood pressure (BP) control

      ii. May be harmful in Prinzmetal's angina and angina from cocaine abuse

    b. Selective β_1 blockers

      i. Atenolol 25 to 100 mg PO daily

      ii. Metoprolol 25 to 200 mg PO BID

  2. ACE-inhibitors

    a. General

      i. Best helps with left ventricle dysfunction, congestive heart failure, and diabetes

    b. Medications

      i. Lisinopril (Zestril) 10 to 40 mg PO daily

      ii. Benazepril (Lotensin) 10 to 40 mg PO daily

IV. Pharmacological management of ACS (*MONA-β*)

  a. *M*orphine for relief of chest pain (eg., Morphine 1 mg IV—titrate to effect)

  b. *O*xygen

  c. *N*itrates (Nitroglycerin SL 0.4 mg q5min × 3; may add Nitro paste; watch BP, as nitro will decrease BP)

  d. *A*spirin 325 mg PO (chewed) STAT (Consider clopidogrel 75 mg PO if patient cannot take aspirin)

---

[a]Remove nitro 10 to 12 hours each day to prevent tolerance

    e. β-blocker IV (eg., Metoprolol 5 mg IV q2min × 3, then 50 mg PO q6h × 2 days, then 100 mg BID)

    f. Heparin drip to achieve prothrombin time (PTT) 1.5–2.5 × control, OR low molecular weight heparin (LMWH), for example, Enoxaparin (Lovenox) 1 mg per kg SC q12h

    g. Consider glycoprotein IIb/IIIa inhibitor for antithrombotic effect

       i. Example—Eptifibatide (Integrilin) 180 μg per kg IV bolus, then infuse at 2 μg/kg/minute

V. Psychiatric pearls, pointers, and parallels

    a. Symptoms of angina are similar to those of a panic attack.

    b. Cardiac complaints need to be taken seriously, particularly in those with cardiac risk factors.

    c. Ask about cocaine use, as this substance places the patient at risk for myocardial infarction.

       i. Avoid β-blockers in treating a cocaine user's chest pain.

2.6

ANTIBIOTIC CROSS-SENSITIVITIES

I. Cross-reactivity

    a. General—a drug never before taken, but with structural similarity to a drug previously taken, may elicit allergic side effects given a preexisting immune response elicited by the previously taken drug.

II. Penicillin and cephalosporin cross-reactivity

    a. Structural similarity—β-lactam ring and similar side chain

    b. Epidemiology—up to 10% of patients with a penicillin allergy have an adverse reaction to cephalosporins.

    c. Medications involved

       i. Penicillins include penicillin, amoxicillin, ampicillin, methicillin, oxacillin, ticarcillin, and so on

       ii. Cephalosporins include cephalexin (Keflex), ceftriaxone (Rocephin), cefaclor (Ceclor), and so on

    d. Recommendations for a patient who has an allergy to either drug

       i. Substitute with a non-β-lactam antimicrobial agent, e.g. Ciprofloxacin may be used for cellulitis.

       ii. If a penicillin or cephalosporin must be used, then

          1. Patient undergoes skin testing to the drug to which he is allegedly allergic.

      a. If negative, then very low risk of immediate adverse reaction.

      b. If positive, consider desensitization to the drug to be used.

III. Sulfonamide cross-reactivity

  a. Structural similarity—SO_2-NH_x is the sulfonamide structure.

    i. Antimicrobial agents—SMX (sulfamethoxazole), sulfadiazine, sulfacetamide

    ii. Non-antimicrobial agents—furosemide (Lasix), celecoxib (Celebrex), sulfonylureas

> **NOTE:**
>
> However, the structure of the antimicrobial agents and the non-antimicrobials noted in the preceding text differs enough such that cross-reactivity between these groups is thought to be unlikely.

IV. Psychiatric pearls, pointers, and parallels

  a. Patients with a history of intravenous drug use are prone to a myriad of infections, ranging from cellulitis to endocarditis.

  b. Maintenance medications for substance abuse, such as methadone, interact with many antibiotics.

    i. Methadone and ciprofloxacin can increase the risk of QT prolongation.

2.7

APHTHOUS ULCERS (CANKER SORES)

I. Evaluation

  a. General—common, painful lesions are present on the labial mucosa or mucous membranes of the oral cavity.

  b. Description—usually red, sometimes have a white coating; not contagious.

> **REMEMBER:**
>
> Aphthous ulcers (canker sores) are different from fever blisters, which are typically found on the outside of one's lips or at the corners of the mouth.

c. Clinical—if benign, the patient should NOT have fever, adenopathy, gastrointestinal (GI) symptoms, or skin manifestations.

d. Etiology—unclear; consequently treatments focus on symptoms rather than a specific cause.

e. Epidemiology—they are more common in young adults (teens–20s).

f. Classification

   i. Minor aphthae—can be singular or multiple, <1 cm in diameter, and shallow

   ii. Major aphthae—diameter is >1 cm and ulceration is deeper; more likely to scar

   iii. Herpetiform aphthae—very numerous and vesicular in nature

---

NOTE:

Benign aphthae are usually smaller and more likely to be self-limited as opposed to more serious conditions (as listed in subsequent text).

II. Differential diagnosis (with diagnostic discriminators noted)

a. Infectious

   i. Viral

      1. Herpes simplex virus (HSV)—vesicular; Tzank stain reveals inclusion-bearing giant cells

      2. Cytomegalovirus (CMV)—biopsy reveals multinucleated giant cells

      3. Varicella (chicken pox/zoster)

      4. Coxsackie virus—may also have hand and foot lesions

   ii. Treponemal

      1. Example: syphilis—rapid plasma reagin (RPR) positive

        a. Psychiatric correlate—neurosyphilis most frequently presents with personality change

   iii. Fungal (e.g., cryptosporidium, mucormycosis, histoplasma—biopsy and culture positive)

b. Autoimmune

   i. Behçet's syndrome—ulceration of genitals, uveitis, iritis, and arthritis

      1. Psychiatric correlate—neurologic involvement (personality change, psychosis) → poor prognosis

   ii. Reiter's syndrome—conjunctivitis, urethritis, arthritis (cannot see, pee, or climb a tree)

   iii. Crohn's disease—inflammatory disease of the entire GI tract with other GI ulcerations

   iv. Lupus erythematosus—antinuclear antibody (ANA) positive, damages multiple organ systems

      1. Psychiatric correlates

        a. Personality change, psychosis, affective disorders, and anxiety may accompany lupus.

        b. Stroke and seizures seen in lupus patients may be implicated in psychiatric phenomena.

        c. Cognitive dysfunction is experienced by up to 50% of patients with lupus.

        d. Central nervous system (CNS) vasculitis is the most severe form of lupus.

            i. Patient may present with high fever, neck stiffness, seizures, and psychosis.

     v. Bullous pemphigoid—generalized bullae (blisters) found throughout the skin

     vi. Pemphigus vulgaris—bullae are localized before they become generalized

  c. Hematologic

     i. Neutropenia

     ii. Neoplasm

III. Treatment

  a. Antibiotic therapy (empiric treatment, some data)

     i. Tetracycline 250 mg per 5 mL "swish and spit" QID × 5 days

  b. Anti-inflammatory agents (beware of potential for fungal infection with steroid rinses)

     i. Triamcinolone (Kenalog) 0.1% in Orabase—apply to dried ulcer BID to QID until healed

     ii. Dexamethasone elixir 0.5 mg per 5 mL "swish and spit" q12h until healed

  c. Other agents

     i. Viscous lidocaine 2%—apply to ulcer several times daily p.r.n.

     ii. Over-the-counter Benzocaine preparations

        1. Anbesol—apply up to 4 times daily.

        2. Zilactin-B—apply up to 4 times daily.

        3. Oragel—apply up to 4 times daily.

     iii. Orabase—apply up to 4 times daily.

2.8

ARRHYTHMIAS

REMEMBER:

With arrhythmias, get vital signs, an electrocardiography (EKG), and a rhythm strip.

I. Supraventricular arrhythmias
   a. Premature atrial complexes (PACs)
      i. General—generated from an atrial ectopic focus; therefore, P wave is different from sinus P wave
      ii. Clinical—typically asymptomatic
      iii. Risk factors—excess caffeine or alcohol, sympathomimetic drugs, structural heart disease
      iv. Treatment—none required; limit risks; β-blocker at low dose if uncomfortable symptoms
   b. Atrial fibrillation (A-fib)
      i. General—atria exhibit disorganized, rapid, irregular activity; the same for the ventricles
      ii. Clinical—EKG shows an irregularly irregular rhythm (see Figure 2.8.1)
         1. May be asymptomatic at rates <100
         2. Likely symptomatic when rapid ventricular response (RVR)
            a. Palpitations, lightheadedness, shortness of breath, weakness
      iii. Etiology (PIRATES)—(Patient may convert to regular rhythm if these causes are treated)
         1. *P*ulmonary disease
         2. *I*schemia
         3. *R*heumatic heart disease
         4. *A*trial myxoma
         5. *T*hyroid, *T*heophylline
         6. *E*thanol
         7. *S*timulants, *S*epsis, *S*urgery
      iv. Epidemiology—3% to 5% of patients older than 60 years; 9% of patients older than 75 years
      v. Risk Factors—hypertension (HTN), left ventricular hypertrophy (LVH), cardiomyopathy, coronary artery disease (CAD), chronic obstructive pulmonary disease (COPD), diabetes mellitus (DM) in ♀
      vi. Rhythm/rate management
         1. Restoration of sinus rhythm in acute onset OR severe compromise from A-fib
            a. If within 48 hours of new onset A-fib—chemical or electric cardioversion
            b. If >48 hours or unknown time, then ↑ chance of atrial thrombi. Get transesophageal echocardiograph
               i. If thrombi, anticoagulate (international normalized ratio [INR] 2–3 for 3 weeks) precardioversion
               ii. If no thrombi, may cardiovert and utilize short-term anticoagulation
         2. Rate control in chronic A-fib OR new-onset A-fib with RVR
            a. Calcium channel blocker (CCB)—Diltiazem 0.25 mg per kg IV over 2 minutes;

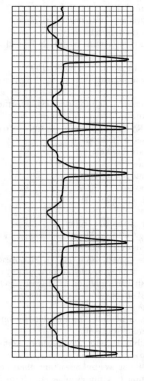

FIGURE 2.8.1 Atrial fibrillation. Courtesy of the author.

then, 0.35 mg per kg after 15 minutes if needed;
then, 10 mg per hour in drip if needed
PO maintenance—Diltiazem (Cardizem) 30 to 90 mg
QID
b. β-Blocker—Metoprolol 2.5 to 5 mg IV over 2 minutes;
may repeat q5min up to a total dose of 15 mg as
needed
PO maintenance—Metoprolol (Lopressor) 25 to
100 mg BID
c. Digoxin 0.25 to 0.5 mg IV;
then, 0.25 mg q4h to q6h to a total of 1.0 mg
PO maintenance—Digoxin (Lanoxin) 0.125 to
0.25 mg daily
   i. Monitor
      1. Serum levels—therapeutic = 0.5 to 1.0 ng
         per mL
      2. Laboratory findings—liver function tests
         (LFTs), electrolytes (K, Mg, Ca), renal func-
         tion, EKG
   ii. Digitalis toxicity
      1. Gastrointestinal (GI) (nausea, vomiting,
         abdominal pain)
      2. Neurologic (confusion, headache)
      3. Cardiovascular (arrhythmia)
      4. Visual disturbances (changes in color per-
         ception, blurred vision, colored halos around
         objects, scotomas—area of diminished vision)
vii. Anticoagulation (for those with persistent A-fib)
   1. Long-term anticoagulation is recommended to reduce
      the risk of stroke.
      a. Risk of stroke is 4.5% per year in patients with A-fib
         and normal valve function.
   2. Risk for thromboembolic events can be measured by
      CHADS2 score.
      a. *C*ongestive heart failure (1 point)
      b. *H*ypertension (1 point)
      c. *A*ge of 75 or older (1 point)
      d. *D*iabetes (1 point)
      e. Prevention in patients with a prior ischemic *S*troke or
         transient ischemic attack (TIA) (2 points)
         Low risk = 0; intermediate risk = 1 to 2; high risk ≥3
   3. Anticoagulate with warfarin (Coumadin) to an INR goal
      of 2 to 3
      a. INR is monitored initially frequently (once a week).
      b. Once level is stable, monitor once every 3 to 4 weeks.
      c. Warfarin is contraindicated in pregnancy.
c. Atrial flutter
   i. Clinical

        1. "Sawtooth" appearance on EKG
        2. Atrial rate of 300 bpm; ventricular rates of 150 bpm (2:1) or 75 bpm (4:1)
    ii. Management—As with A-fib, get back to sinus rhythm and maintain it; may need ablation.

  d. Paroxysmal supraventricular tachycardias (PSVT)

    i. Mechanisms
        1. Atrioventricular nodal reentry tachycardia (AVNRT)
          a. Clinical—EKG shows a narrow-complex QRS with no evident P waves.
        2. Accessory pathways causing PSVT
            For example, Wolf-Parkinson-White syndrome (WPW, pre-excitation syndrome)
          a. Clinical—EKG shows a short PR interval and "delta wave."
        3. Increased automaticity causing PSVT
          a. Clinical—multiple foci in the atria fire producing varying P waves

    ii. Management
        1. If hemodynamically unstable—electric cardioversion
        2. If stable
          a. Nonpharmacologic
            i. Vagal maneuvers
              1. Increase parasympathetic tone
              2. Decrease atrioventricular (AV) node conduction
            ii. Avoid inciting factors
              1. Caffeine, tobacco, EtOH, medications, stress
          b. Pharmacologic
            i. Slow or block AV nodal conduction
              1. Adenosine (ultra short-acting), CCB, β-blocker, and so on

---

REMEMBER:

In general, avoid AV nodal blockers with WPW as well as undiagnosed wide-complex QRS tachycardia; these can degenerate into ventricular fibrillation (V-fib).

---

          c. Ablation
          d. Electronic pacing

  e. Sinus arrhythmia
    i. General—normal event in young people that is usually asymptomatic
    ii. Clinical—EKG → RR interval shortens during inspiration and lengthens during expiration
    iii. Treatment—typically unnecessary

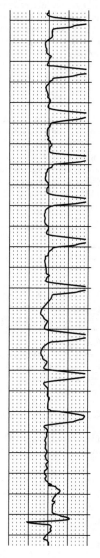

FIGURE 2.8.2 Ventricular tachycardia. Courtesy of the author.

II. Ventricular arrhythmias
   a. Premature ventricular complexes (PVCs)
      i. Clinical—premature occurrence of a wide QRS complex
      ii. Epidemiology—more prevalent with older age
      iii. Risk factors—structural heart disease, metabolic ($\uparrow\downarrow$ K, $\downarrow$ Mg, hypoxemia), stimulants (cocaine, amphetamines, caffeine), sympathomimetic drugs (over-the-counter cold preparations, and so on)
      iv. Treatment—usually none required; correct risks; β-blocker if symptoms severe, disabling

> **NOTE:**
>
> "Ventricular bigeminy" = alternating sinus beats and PVCs.

   b. Ventricular tachycardia (VT)
      i. General—ventricular ectopic focus is the source of VT.
      ii. Clinical—EKG shows wide-complex tachycardia (three or more successive PVCs) (see Figure 2.8.2).
         1. Rate >100 bpm
         2. No associated P waves

> **REMEMBER:**
>
> VT is assumed for any wide-complex tachycardia until proven otherwise.

      iii. Management
         1. If hemodynamically unstable—electric cardioversion
         2. If stable
            a. Antiarrhythmic agents such as Amiodarone
            b. Automatic implantable cardioverter-defibrillators (ICDs)
            c. Ventricular fibrillation (V-fib)
               i. Medical emergency → Defibrillate!
III. Psychiatric pearls, pointers, and parallels
   a. Symptoms of arrhythmias can be similar to those of a panic attacks.
   b. Tricyclic antidepressants can cause arrhythmias and may be cardiotoxic.
   c. Lithium can cause hyperthyroidism, which in turn can induce arrhythmias such as A-fib.

ASTHMA

I. Evaluation
   a. Description—a chronic disorder of the airways characterized by
      i. Variable airflow obstruction (usually reversible with treatment or spontaneously)
      ii. Bronchial hyper-responsiveness
      iii. Airway inflammation related to immunologically mediated (e.g., immunoglobulin E [IgE]) responses
   b. Clinical—shortness of breath, wheezing, chest tightness, cough (dry or productive)
   c. Epidemiology—affects approximately 15 million Americans; 1.5 million emergency room (ER) visits each year
   d. Risk factors—genetic (atopy) and environmental (exposures, allergens, viruses) factors
   e. Classification (National Asthma Education and Prevention Program [NAEPP]) (see Table 2.9.1)

NOTE:

Inhalation of β_2-agonists delivered through a metered dose inhaler (MDI) using proper technique is just as effective as a nebulizer.

II. Treatment specifics
   a. β_2-agonists
      i. Short-acting (for p.r.n. therapy)
         1. Albuterol (Ventolin/Proventil) two puffs inhaled q4h p.r.n.
      ii. Long-acting (for maintenance therapy, not to be used acutely)
         1. Salmeterol (Serevent Diskus) 50 μg inhaled q12h
   b. Inhaled corticosteroids
      i. Fluticasone (Flovent HFA) 88 to 440 μg inhaled BID
      ii. Beclomethasone (QVAR) 40 to 160 μg inhaled BID
   c. Combined β_2-agonists and inhaled corticosteroids
      i. Fluticasone/salmeterol (Advair Diskus) [100, 250, or 500]/50 μg inhaled q12h
   d. Cromolyn sodium (Intal)
      i. For chronic asthma—two puffs inhaled QID
      ii. For exercise-induced asthma—two puffs inhaled 10 to 60 minutes preexercise
   e. Theophylline (Theolair, Theo-24 [sustained release version])

TABLE 2.9.1 National Asthma Education and Prevention Program (NAEPP) Classification

	Activity	Daytime Symptoms	Nighttime Symptoms	Lung Function	Quick Relief	Long-term Control
Mild intermittent	Normal between exacerbations	$\leq 2 \times$/wk	$\leq 2 \times$/mo	FEV_1 or PEF >80% predicted; PEF variability <20%	Short-acting β_2-agonist MDI p.r.n.	No medicines, but educate patient
Exercise-induced	—	—	—		Preexercise: Short-acting β_2-agonist MDI OR cromolyn	Inhaled corticosteroid
Mild persistent	May be affected by exacerbations	>2 ×/wk	>2 ×/mo	FEV_1 or PEF $\geq$80% predicted; PEF variability 20%–30%	Short-acting β_2-agonist MDI p.r.n.	Low-dose inhaled corticosteroid Alternatives: Cromolyn, theophylline low-dose, OR leukotriene receptor antagonist
Moderate persistent	Activity affected by exacerbations	Daily	>1 ×/wk	FEV_1 or PEF 61%–79% predicted; PEF variability >30%	Short-acting β_2-agonist MDI p.r.n.	Medium-dose inhaled corticosteroid and long-acting β_2-agonist MDI p.r.n. Alternative additions: Theophylline OR leukotriene receptor antagonist
Severe persistent	Physical activity limited	Continual	Frequent	FEV_1 or PEF $\leq$60% predicted; PEF variability >30%	Short-acting β_2-agonist MDI p.r.n.	High-dose inhaled corticosteroid and long-acting β_2-agonist MDI p.r.n. Consider adding: Oral corticosteroid

FEV_1, forced expiratory volume in one second; PEF, peak expiratory flow; MDI, metered dose inhaler.

(Adapted from National Asthma Education and Prevention Program. Expert panel report: Guidelines for the diagnosis and management of asthma update on selected topics—2002. *J Allergy Clin Immunol.* 2002;110:S141–S219 and Naureckas ET, Solway J. Mild Asthma. *N Engl J Med.* 2001;345(17):1257–1262.)

      i. Initially—10 mg per kg of body weight per day PO (divided TID–QID for regular formulation)

      ii. Maintenance—6 to 8 mg per kg of body weight/day; not to exceed 400 mg per day

         1. But, can be gradually increased to 13 mg per kg, not to exceed 900 mg per day.

         2. And, monitor serum levels. Therapeutic theophylline is 10 to 20 μg per mL.

            a. Some patients respond to levels of 5 to 10 μg per mL

            b. Many prefer levels 10 to 15 μg per mL

            c. Levels >20 typically have gastrointestinal (GI) (nausea, intractable vomiting), cardiac (arrhythmias), neurologic side effects (headaches, status epilepticus)

    f. Leukotriene receptor antagonists

      i. Montelukast (Singulair) 10 mg PO qhs

      ii. Zafirlukast (Accolate) 20 mg PO BID (hepatotoxicity occurs in rare instances)

    g. Oral corticosteroids—for initial relief in severe cases

      i. Prednisone 40 mg per day, tapering to 0 over 2 weeks

III. Prevention

    a. Patient education

      i. Make sure the patient can recognize and manage flares and identify triggers.

      ii. Make sure the patient understands how to use medications (i.e., how to use an MDI).

    b. Patient monitoring

      i. Have patient see his primary care physician (PCP) or pulmonologist at least every 6 months even if mild symptoms

      ii. Objective measures—spirometry preferred over peak-flow assessment

IV. Psychiatric pearls, pointers, and parallels

    a. Treatment for asthma, chronic obstructive pulmonary disease (COPD), and a host of other inflammatory conditions often includes steroids

      i. Psychiatric manifestations of steroid use (whether started acutely or used in chronic treatment) include:

         1. Mental status changes (cognitive impairment, delirium, psychosis)

         2. Affective symptoms (mood lability, depression, mania/hypomania, agitation, irritability)

         3. Anxiety

      ii. Steroid-induced psychosis can be treated with neuroleptics.

         1. Most patients recover completely with appropriate treatment and cessation of steroid.

      iii. The combination of tricyclic antidepressants (TCAs) and steroids can worsen outcome.

   1. In those treated with TCAs, affective and psychotic symptoms can worsen even after the steroid has been tapered off.
    iv. A history of a psychiatric disorder does not clearly increase the risk of developing a psychotic reaction.
     v. A history of steroid-induced psychopathology does not predict response to prednisone in the future.

2.10

BRONCHITIS (ACUTE)

I. Evaluation
   a. Description—"chest cold" in a patient without underlying cardiopulmonary disease lasting <3 weeks
   b. Clinical
      i. Main symptoms—cough within 2 days of infection and lasting 2 to 8 weeks, ± phlegm production

> **NOTE:**
>
> Purulence is from peroxidase released by white blood cells (WBCs); therefore, sputum color alone is NOT an indication of bacterial infection.

      ii. Additional symptoms—shortness of breath, wheezing, chest pain, fever, malaise, and hoarseness
   c. Mechanism—bronchial injury → inflammation → airway hyperresponsiveness and mucus production
   d. Etiology
      i. Viral (most cases)—during influenza season, perform rapid influenza testing
      ii. Bacterial (5% of cases)—most common—*Mycoplasma, Bordetella*, and *Chlamydia*
      iii. Yeast and fungi
      iv. Noninfectious (asthma, air pollutants, cannabis, tobacco, etc.)
   e. Imaging—no need for chest x-ray (CXR) in acute bronchitis
      i. CXR only for those whose examination suggests pneumonia or cardiopulmonary disease
II. Differential diagnosis
   a. Asthma

b. Upper respiratory tract infection
c. Pneumonia

REMEMBER:

If fever >38°C, heart rate (HR) >100, respiration rate (RR) >24, and/or consolidation on lung examination → suspect pneumonia!

III. Treatment
   a. Expectorants (promote expulsion of phlegm)
      i. Guaifenesin 200 to 400 mg PO q4h
      ii. Guaifenesin SR (Mucinex) 600 mg q12h p.r.n.
      iii. For patients with diabetes mellitus, consider sugar-free, alcohol-free Diabetic Tussin EX (guaifenesin)
   b. Antitussives (control or prevent cough; indicated if cough is creating significant discomfort.)
      i. Nonopioid
         1. Dextromethorphan (may be referred to as *DM*) 10 to 20 mg PO q4h
         2. Benzonatate (Tessalon Pearls) 100 to 200 mg PO TID
      ii. Opioid
         1. Codeine 10 to 20 mg PO q4h (take with food)
   c. Antitussive/expectorant combination
      i. Codeine/guaifenesin (Robitussin AC) 10/300 PO q4h
   d. Bronchodilators (β_2-agonists)
      i. Albuterol (Proventil) two puffs inhaled q4h
   e. Antibiotics
      i. Not indicated for patients (including smokers) unless underlying cardiopulmonary disease
      ii. Antibiotic regimens that have been utilized
         1. Azithromycin (Zithromax) 500 mg PO daily × 3 days
         2. Trimethoprim-sulfamethoxazole (Bactrim) 160/800 mg PO q12h × 7 to 10 days
         3. Amoxicillin (Amoxil) 500 mg PO q8h × 7 to 10 days
         4. Amoxicillin/clavulanate 500/125 (Augmentin) PO q8h × 7 to 10 days
         5. Doxycycline (Vibramycin) 100 mg PO q12h × 7 to 10 days
   f. If symptoms are associated with allergic rhinitis, then treat as such (see Chapter 2.2).
   g. Encourage rest and fluids
   h. Vaporizers and humidifiers may provide symptomatic relief

---

NOTE:

If symptoms persist for >2 weeks despite appropriate treatment, reevaluate—consider CXR, pulmonary function tests (PFTs), peak flow measurement, sputum culture, and antibiotic therapy.

BURNS

I. Classification
   a. The traditional classification (first, second, or third degree) is being replaced by a system based on depth (see Table 2.11.1).
II. Acute management
   a. After establishing classification based on depth, determine extent of burn.
      i. "Rule of Nines"—divides the surface area (SA) of the body into multiples of 9%.
         1. One percent SA—perineum (1% total)
         2. Each = 9% SA—total head, total left arm, total right arm (27% total)
         3. Each = 9% SA—front left leg, back left leg, front right leg, back right leg (36% total)

TABLE 2.11.1 Burn Classification Based on Depth

	Depth of Affected Area	Cause	Appearance	Sensation
Superficial	Epidermis	UV radiation from sun Very short flame exposure	Erythematous Blanches with pressure No blisters Dry surface	Painful (usually delayed for several hours after sun exposure)
Superficial partial-thickness	Epidermis + superficial dermis	Short flame exposure Scald from a spill or splash	Erythematous Blanches with pressure, BUT slow capillary refill Thin-walled blisters Moist, moderate edema	Extremely painful, particularly when blisters break Even painful to air and temperature
Deep partial-thickness	Epidermis + deep dermis	Flame exposure Scald from spill Hot oil, grease	Red or waxy white May NOT blanch Blisters usually absent Moist, wet, marked edema	Sensation is altered May only perceive pressure
Full-thickness	Epidermis + dermis + subcutaneous tissue, muscle, bone	Fame exposure Scaled from immersion Hot oil, grease, and chemicals High voltage	Waxy white to black Does NOT blanch Fluid shifts—edema	Sensation is altered May only perceive deep pressure

UV, ultraviolet.
(Adapted from Morgan ED, Bledsoe SC, Barker J. Ambulatory management of burns. *Am Fam Physician.* 2000;62(9):2015–2029.)

TABLE 2.11.2   Grading for Burn Severity

	Criteria	Disposition
Minor burn	<10% SA burn in an adult OR <2% full-thickness burn	Outpatient management
Moderate burn	10%–20% SA burn in an adult OR 2%–5% full-thickness burn OR burn + medical problem predisposing to infection	Hospital admission
Major burn	>20% SA burn in an adult OR >5% full-thickness burn OR burn + known inhalation injury OR facial/genital injury	Hospital admission— burn center

SA, surface area.

(Adapted from American Burn Association. Hospital and prehospital resources for optimal care of patients with burn injury: guidelines for development and operation of burn centers. *J Burn Care Rehabil.* 1990;11:98–104.)

4. Each = 18% SA—front of chest/abdomen, upper and lower back (36% total)
   b. Grading for burn severity and disposition (see Table 2.11.2).
   c. Hospital admission may require treatment in the intensive care unit (ICU) due to compromised airway, hemodynamic instability, and other trauma that may accompany the burn injury.
III. Ambulatory treatment for minor burns (6 C's)
   a. *C*lothing—remove promptly except for adherent clothing (which is removed in cleaning phase).
   b. *C*ooling—use a sterile saline soaked gauze at 50°F to 55°F to cool the affected area.
   c. *C*leaning—critical phase, but can cause excruciating pain (so establish local/regional anesthesia).
      i. Disinfectants are widely used, but generally discouraged as they can inhibit healing.
      ii. Wash burns with mild soap and tap water, then thoroughly rinse.
   d. *C*hemoprophylaxis
      i. Tetanus prophylaxis—given even for small partial-thickness burns (see Chapter 2.59)
      ii. Infected burn (lymphangitis, fever, malaise, etc.)—hospitalize for IV antibiotics
      iii. Topical prophylaxis (not necessarily needed for superficial burns)—used to prevent infections
         1. Silver sulfadiazine (Silvadene) applied topically daily or BID.
            a. Do NOT use on face or in patients with sulfonamide hypersensitivity.
            b. Do NOT use in pregnant women, newborns, or nursing mothers.

   2. Bacitracin applied topically BID to TID.
    a. May be used instead of Silvadene for superficial partial-thickness burns.
   3. Biologic dressings—decrease infection and increase healing, but expensive and hard to apply.
  e. Covering—acts as a barrier to infection and keeps wound dry.
   i. Not required in superficial burns; instead, may use skin lubricant (e.g., aloe vera cream).
   ii. Cover partial and full-thickness burns with sterile dressings typically BID and then decrease frequency.
    1. Therefore, clean the burn → apply a thin layer of topical antibiotic → apply dressing
  f. Comforting—provide analgesics for pain control.
   i. Avoid aspirin products as they cause platelet inhibition and thereby increase the risk of bleeding.

IV. Psychiatric pearls, pointers, and parallels
 a. Psychiatry is often consulted to see burn victims in the ICU for numerous reasons
  i. The patient is delirious secondary to high doses of narcotics or benzodiazepines used for comfort.
   1. Treat delirium with low-dose antipsychotics
    a. Given the potential for a compromised cardiac status in burn victims, check an EKG.
  ii. The patient is delirious secondary to substance withdrawal.
   1. Watch for alcohol or other drug withdrawal syndromes in these patients.
  iii. A psychiatric diagnosis may have precipitated the burn injury.
   1. Burn injuries due to accidental trauma
    a. For example—an intoxicated patient accidentally burns himself after falling asleep with a cigarette.
   2. Burn injuries due to intentional self-injury possibly with the goal of committing suicide
 b. In all cases, obtain collateral information regarding psychiatric history and medications the patient may be taking.

CANDIDIASIS— MUCOCUTANEOUS INFECTIONS

I. Candidiasis (most common opportunistic fungal infection)
   a. General—ranges from localized mucocutaneous infection to life-threatening disseminated infection
   b. Etiology
      i. *Candida albicans* is the most common.
      ii. Other common culpable candida species include glabrata, parapsilosis, and tropicalis.
   c. Mechanism
      i. *C. albicans* is a normal commensal organism of the oral cavity.
      ii. Candidiasis develops when the host is impaired and *Candida* is able to overgrow.
   d. Risk factors
      i. Impaired salivary gland function from medical problems, medications, or radiotherapy
      ii. Inhaled/PO steroids (and Cushing's) that may suppress cellular immunity and phagocytosis
      iii. Broad-spectrum antibiotics that change the local flora
      iv. Immunosuppressed states such as human immunodeficiency virus (HIV) and malignancy (e.g., leukemia)
      v. Antineoplastic agents and those with neutropenia
      vi. Diabetes, high-carbohydrate diet
      vii. Smoking
      viii. Dentures (which produce an environment conducive to *Candida*'s growth)
      ix. Nutritional deficiencies
      x. Extremes of life
II. Classification of oral candidiasis (most common human fungal infection)
   a. Acute candidiasis
      i. Acute pseudomembranous candidiasis (thrush)
         1. Clinical—white patches throughout oral cavity (mucosa, palate, tongue) which can typically be scraped off to reveal erythematous, nonulcerated mucosa.
         2. Differential diagnosis—lichen planus, squamous cell carcinoma, leukoplakia
      ii. Acute atrophic candidiasis
         1. Clinical—burning sensation in the mouth; may have glossitis

b. Chronic candidiasis
  i. Chronic hyperplastic candidiasis (candidal leukoplakia)
      1. Clinical—buccal mucosa or lateral aspect of the tongue with white lesions
      2. Risk factors—smoking; complete resolution is dependent on smoking cessation
  ii. Chronic atrophic candidiasis (denture stomatitis)
      1. Clinical—localized chronic erythema of those tissues covered by dentures
      2. Risk factors—dentures
  iii. Median rhomboid glossitis
      1. Clinical—affects symmetric area anterior to circumvallate papillae of tongue
      2. Risk factors—smoking, inhaled steroids
c. Angular cheilitis (stomatitis)
  i. Clinical—painful, red fissuring at one or two corners of the mouth
  ii. Treatment—antifungal steroid creams/ointments
III. Management of oral candidiasis
  a. Pharmacologic
    i. Topical
        1. Clotrimazole troche 10 mg PO five times per day × 14 days
        2. Nystatin 5 mL (500,000 units) PO QID—use for 48 hours after symptoms resolve
    ii. Systemic
        1. Fluconazole 200 mg PO or IV on day 1, then 100 mg daily × 13 days
    iii. Consider prophylaxis
        1. Clotrimazole troche 10 mg PO TID
  b. Nonpharmacologic
    i. Regular oral hygiene
    ii. Limit risk factors if possible
IV. Other nonsystemic candidal infections
  a. Candidal esophagitis
    i. Clinical—odynophagia; may accompany oral candidiasis or occur independently
    ii. Risk factors—nearly always related to immune dysfunction (e.g., acquired immunodeficiency syndrome (AIDS) with low CD4)
    iii. Treatment—fluconazole 200 mg PO or IV on day 1, then 100 mg daily × 13 days
  b. Candidal vulvovaginitis (see Chapter 2.58)
    i. Clinical—pruritus, vaginal discomfort, curd-like discharge, painful coitus; white plaques on vaginal walls
    ii. Risk factors—Diabetes mellitus, antibiotics, steroids, HIV, ↑ estrogen levels (oral contraceptive pills, pregnancy)
    iii. Treatment—fluconazole 150 mg PO × 1 dose

   c. Cutaneous candidiasis
       i. Clinical
           1. Erythematous, pruritic, (sometimes) pustular lesions with
               a distinct border
           2. Nearly always associated with satellite lesions (which dis-
               tinguishes it from tinea)
           3. Mostly in intertriginous areas
       ii. Treatment—Nystatin topical cream (or powder if very moist
            area) BID to TID

2.13

CEREBROVASCULAR DISEASE: TRANSIENT ISCHEMIC ATTACK AND STROKE

I. Cerebrovascular disease (CVD)
    a. General—disorders affecting part of the brain transiently or
        permanently by ischemia or bleeding
    b. Classification
        i. Transient ischemic attack (TIA)
            1. Brief neurologic deficit caused by brain ischemia typically
                lasting <1 hour
                a. After a TIA, the 90-day risk of stroke is approxi-
                    mately 10%.
            2. Differential diagnosis of a TIA—stroke, seizure, syncope,
                or migraine
        ii. Stroke
            1. A neurologic deficit involving a particular distribution
                which lasts >24 hours
                a. Types
                    i. Ischemic stroke (85% of strokes)
                        1. Thrombotic (most common)
                            a. Risk factors—hypertension, diabetes,
                                atherosclerosis, and so on
                        2. Embolic
                            a. Risk factors—atrial fibrillation, valve dis-
                                ease, and so on
                    ii. Hemorrhagic stroke (15% of strokes)
                        1. Subarachnoid hemorrhage (SAH)
                        2. Intracerebral hemorrhage

NOTE:
At the time of the incident, there is no way to determine if the ischemia will be a TIA or stroke.

II. Evaluation
   a. Clinical—presentation is contingent on the cerebral vessel involved. (Table 2.13.1)
   b. Imaging
      i. Noncontrast head CT to rule out cerebral hemorrhage or mass lesion and aid in diagnosis.
      ii. Brain magnetic resonance imaging (MRI) may not identify hemorrhage.
         1. However diffusion-weighted imaging (DWI) modality of MRI detects lesion 15 minutes after onset.
   c. Management
      i. Thrombolysis with tissue plasminogen activator (tPA)
         1. Indication—for those who present within 180 minutes of onset of symptoms (Table 2.13.2)
      ii. Blood pressure control
         1. Within the first 24 hours of a TIA or stroke, do not treat blood pressure, unless >220/120
            a. Exceptions—hypertensive crisis, end organ compromise, dissection, and so on

TABLE 2.13.1 Presentation of Neurologic Consequences in Cerebrovascular Disease

Involved Artery	Neurologic Consequence
Middle cerebral artery (MCA)	Hemiplegia (upper extremity and face greater than lower extremity)
	Hemisensory loss
	Homonymous hemianopia
	Aphasia (when dominant hemisphere is involved)
Anterior cerebral artery (ACA)	Hemiplegia (lower extremity greater than upper extremity and face)
	Primitive reflexes
Vertebral and basilar arteries	Ipsilateral cranial nerve findings and cerebellar findings
	Contralateral motor and sensory loss
Lacunar infarction of deep penetrating branches (as seen in elderly hypertensive patients and those with diabetes)	May have motor hemiplegia, sensory loss, ataxia, or dysarthria

Modified from Ferri FF. *Practical guide to the care of the medical patient.* 6th ed. Mosby; 2004:725–739.

TABLE 2.13.2 Criteria for Management of Thrombolysis

Inclusion Criteria	Exclusion Criteria
Ischemic stroke with persistent neurologic deficit	Hemorrhagic stroke or large infarct
≥18 years old	History of intracranial hemorrhage, AV malformation, or aneurysm
	LP or arterial puncture at noncompressible site within ≤1 week
	Serious trauma or major surgery within ≤2 weeks
	GI or urinary tract hemorrhage within ≤3 weeks
	Serious head trauma or stroke within ≤3 months
	History of seizure at stroke onset
	Blood pressure >185/110 (but one can lower blood pressure pre-tPA)
	Glucose <50 mg/dL or >400 mg/dL
	Platelets <100 K
	Heparin within ≤48 hours and elevated PTT OR ... INR >1.5
	Pregnancy

AV, atriovenous; LP, lumbar puncture; GI, gastrointestinal; tPA, tissue plasminogen activator; PTT, partial thromboplastin time; INR, international normalized ratio.
Modified from Goldman L, Bennett JC, eds. *Cecil textbook of medicine*, 21st ed. Philadelphia: WB Saunders; 2000.

2. Pharmacologic treatment
   a. Nonthrombolytic candidates (goal = lower diastolic blood pressure [DBP] by 10%–20%)
      i. DBP >140—nitroprusside (Nitropress) 0.5 μg/kg/min IV
      ii. DBP >120—Labetalol 10 to 20 mg IV over 2 minutes q20min
   b. Thrombolytic candidate
      i. Pre-tPA with DBP >110—Nitropaste 1 to 2 in.
         1. Blood pressure should be <185/110 before giving tPA.
      ii. Post-tPA ... Similar to nonthrombolytic candidates
iii. Antiplatelet therapy—initiate quickly if patient is not a tPA candidate; options include:
   1. Aspirin 81 to 325 mg PO daily
   2. Clopidogrel (Plavix) 75 mg PO daily
      a. The drug is given for those intolerant to aspirin OR on aspirin during an event.
      b. Adverse effects—neutropenia and thrombocytopenic purpura are rare.
   3. Aspirin 25 mg/dipyridamole 200 extended release (ER) (Aggrenox)—one capsule PO BID

        a. For those who would benefit from thrombotic stroke risk reduction

  iv. Long-term risk reduction strategy

    1. Blood pressure (goal: <140/90; unless diabetic or renal disease, <130/80)

      a. Elevated blood pressure is the no.1 treatable risk factor for stroke.

      b. However, abrupt decrease of blood pressure quickly after a stroke can promote ischemia.

    2. Smoking—stroke risk is 50% higher in smokers than nonsmokers.

    3. Heart disease—left ventricular hypertrophy (LVH), atrial fibrillation, arteriovenous (AV) conduction abnormalities, and so on, increases risk.

    4. Lipids—high cholesterol likely increases risk for ischemic stroke (goal: low-density lipoprotein (LDL) <100).

    5. Diabetes—increases the risk of stroke by 25% to 50% (goal: fasting blood sugar <126 mg/dL).

    6. Diet (decrease weight), exercise (increase activity), and alcohol consumption (decrease intake).

    7. Carotid disease—consider carotid endarterectomy for 70% to 99% vessel occlusion.

    8. Anticoagulation—needed for those with high-risk cardioembolic conditions.

      a. Long-term international normalized ratio (INR) goals utilizing warfarin (Coumadin) PO therapy

        i. Mechanical valve = 3.0 to 4.0

        ii. Nonvalvular A-fib = 2.0 to 3.0

        iii. LV thrombus = 2.0 to 3.0 (6 months)

REMEMBER:

Except for those patients with cardioembolic conditions, anticoagulation with warfarin has no greater benefit over antiplatelet therapy and carries greater risk for bleeding.

III. Hemorrhagic stroke

  a. Subarachnoid hemorrhage

    i. General—bleeding into the subarachnoid space usually from trauma, aneurysm, or AV malformation.

    ii. Clinical—abrupt onset of a severe headache radiating to the neck, "worst" headache of one's life.

    iii. Imaging—noncontrast head CT shows blood in basal cisterns or intracerebrally.

    iv. Further tests—lumbar puncture (LP) (after papilledema is ruled out) is grossly bloody with xanthochromia.

    v. Management—(depends on patient's clinical status and if surgical options are feasible.)

1. Medical management
   a. Airway, breathing, circulation (ABCs)
   b. Bed rest, limit stress (stool softeners, stress ulcer prophylaxis, etc.)
   c. Mannitol (Osmitrol)—to reduce cerebral edema
   d. Nimodipine (Nimotop)—to treat cerebral blood vessel spasm
      i. Nimodipine 60 mg PO q4h × 21 days
   e. Fludrocortisone—mineralcorticoid used if patient is hyponatremic
   f. Blood pressure (goal: mean arterial pressure [MAP] ≤125)
      i. If MAP >125, then consider:
         1. Esmolol (Brevibloc) 500 μg per kg over 1 minute IV
            OR Enalaprilat (Vasotec IV) 1 to 5 mg IV.

NOTE:

Roughly, MAP = 1/3 systolic blood pressure (SBP) + 2/3 DBP

---

2. Surgical management—(for aneurysms)
   a. Whether to implement clipping or endovascular coiling depends on aneurysm size, patient's age and condition, and neurosurgeon's expertise.
b. Intracerebral hemorrhage
   i. General—bleeding within the deep structures of the brain
   ii. Clinical—typically occurs during periods of activity; headache and neurologic deficits seen (Table 2.13.3)
   iii. Etiology—hypertension (50%–60%), hemorrhagic infarcts, anticoagulant use, tumors, and so on
   iv. Imaging—noncontrast head CT shows hemorrhage
   v. Management
      1. Medical management
         a. Airway, breathing, circulation (ABCs), intensive care unit (ICU) care
         b. Increased intracranial pressure (ICP)
            i. Mannitol (Osmitrol)—titrate to serum osmolarity of 300
            ii. Mechanical ventilation to prevent hypoxia and hypercapnia
               1. Stimulates cerebral vasodilation.
         c. Blood pressure—consider reduction if >180/100
            i. Nitroprusside (Nitropress) IV—titrate to effect
         d. Correct coagulation abnormalities; maintain platelets >50 K
      2. Surgical management
         a. Consider evacuation of hematomas for patients. . .

TABLE 2.13.3   Clinical Aspects of Intracerebral Hemorrhage

Location of Hemorrhage	Eye Movements	Pupils	Additional Neurologic Deficits
Putamen	Eyes look toward the side of the lesion	Normal in size and reactive	Contralateral hemiplegia
Thalamus	Eyes look downward and inward at the nose	Small in size and nonreactive	Contralateral hemisensory loss
Pons	Eyes maintain the midposition; no doll's eye movements	Pinpoint, but reactive	Flaccid quadriplegia Coma is common
Cerebellum	Eyes are unable to look toward the side of the lesion	Normal in size and reactive	Inability to stand or walk Vertigo and dysarthria present

Note: Additionally, signs of increased intracranial pressure may be present (bradycardia, hypoventilation, third nerve palsy).
Modified from Ferri FF. *Practical guide the care of the medical patient,* 6th ed. Mosby; 2004:725–739.

  i. who are noncomatose and have a cerebellar hemorrhage
  ii. with accessible hematomas producing temporal lobe herniation
IV. Psychiatric pearls, pointers, and parallels
 a. Sympathomimetic drugs, such as cocaine, can cause a TIA.

2.14

CHRONIC OBSTRUCTIVE PULMONARY DISEASE

I. Evaluation
 a. General—progressive airflow limitation secondary to chronic inflammation of the lung and airways
  i. This process that destroys the lung results in emphysema, chronic bronchitis, or both.

  1. Emphysema—disease of small airways and alveoli with mucous gland hyperplasia
  2. Chronic bronchitis—cough and sputum on most days for ≥ 3 months over 2 years

  b. Clinical—productive cough, $\pm$ wheezing, dyspnea, accelerated $\downarrow$ in FEV_1, and hyperinflated lungs

---

REMEMBER:

Unlike asthma, which also features airflow obstruction and inflammation, chronic obstructive pulmonary disease (COPD) does not demonstrate reversibility on pulmonary function tests (PFTs); COPD has an incomplete response to β_2-agonists, and airways typically do not demonstrate hyperresponsiveness.

---

  c. Mechanism—not fully understood, but perhaps due to chronic inflammation from inhaled irritants
  d. Epidemiology—approximately 20% of adult Americans have COPD
  e. Risk factors—irritants such as smoking; 90% of cases with smoking as their cause
  f. Staging (as per the Global Initiative for Chronic Obstructive Lung Disease [GOLD]) (see Table 2.14.1)
II. Management of chronic obstructive pulmonary disease exacerbations
  a. Clinical—worsening dyspnea, more purulent and increased sputum production
  b. Etiology—infectious (most often), environmental irritants, congestive heart failure, noncompliance with medications
    i. Common infectious causes
      1. *Streptococcus pneumoniae*, *Haemophilus influenzae*, and *Moraxella catarrhalis* (60% of exacerbations)
      2. Atypical organisms (e.g., *Chlamydia pneumoniae*) (10% of exacerbations)
      3. Viruses (25%–30% of exacerbations)

TABLE 2.14.1 Chronic Obstructive Pulmonary Disease (COPD) Staging

	FEV_1 (%)	Symptoms
Stage I (mild)	≥ 80	Variable symptoms
Stage II (moderate)	50–79	Mild-moderate symptoms
Stage III (severe)	30–49	Symptoms that limit exertion
Stage IV (very severe)	<30	Symptoms that limit daily activities

For COPD, FEV_1/FVC <0.70 on spirometry.
Adapted from Sutherland ER, Cherniack RM. Management of chronic obstructive pulmonary disease. *N Engl J Med.* 2004;350(26):2689–2697.

      4. Severe exacerbations with *Pseudomonas* species and gram-negative rods (GNR).

  c. Treatment

    i. Oxygenation—maintain oxygen saturation $\geq 90\%$ (therefore Pao_2 60–65 mm Hg).

    ii. Inhaled bronchodilators—use nebulizer; proper metered dose inhaler (MDI) use is difficult in an exacerbation.

      1. β_2-agonist (Albuterol) and anticholinergic (Ipratropium) nebulizer q4h

      2. As exacerbation lessens, consider Combivent (albuterol–ipratropium) MDI q4h

    iii. Antibiotics

      1. For mild-moderate exacerbations (which could be managed as an outpatient)

        a. Doxycycline 100 mg PO BID × 10 days
OR TMP-SMZ (Bactrim DS) 1 tablet PO BID × 10 days
OR Amoxicillin-clavulanate (Augmentin) 875/125 PO BID × 10 days

      2. Patients older than 65 years or with more than four exacerbations per year, consider

        a. Azithromycin (Zithromax) 500 mg PO daily × 3 days
OR moxifloxacin (Avelox) 400 mg PO daily × 10 days

      3. For moderate-severe exacerbations (need hospitalization)

        a. Ceftriaxone (Rocephin) 1 to 2 g IV daily

        b. Piperacillin-tazobactam (Zosyn) 3.375 g IV q6h

      4. For severe exacerbations with *Pseudomonas* or GNR (need hospitalization)

        a. Third generation cephalosporin (Ceftriaxone) OR augmented penicillin (Zosyn) + Fluroquinolone (Moxifloxacin) OR Aminoglycoside (Tobramycin)

    iv. Corticosteroids

      1. Methylprednisolone 60 to 125 mg IV q6h to q12h (for 2–3 days in severe exacerbations)

      2. Then, prednisone 60 mg PO daily initially, and tapered over a 2-week period

III. Management of stable chronic obstructive pulmonary disease

  a. Health care maintenance

    i. Smoking cessation—decreases the rate of decline in lung-function

    ii. Vaccination—pneumococcal vaccination and annual influenza vaccination

  b. Pharmacotherapy

    i. Inhaled bronchodilators

      1. Anticholinergics (may provide greater bronchodilation than β_2-agonists)

        a. Short-acting (for p.r.n. therapy)

           i. Ipratropium (Atrovent) two puffs inhaled q4h
               p.r.n.
        b. Long-acting
           i. Tiotropium (Spiriva) one inhalation daily
      2. β_2-agonists
        a. Short-acting (for p.r.n. therapy)
           i. Albuterol (Ventolin/Proventil) two puffs inhaled
               q4h p.r.n.
        b. Long-acting (for maintenance therapy; not to be used
            acutely)
           i. Salmeterol (Serevent Diskus) 50 μg inhaled q12h
    ii. Inhaled corticosteroids (Fluticasone [Flovent HFA]
         88–440 μg inhaled BID)
      1. Little physiologic improvement, but may alleviate symp-
          toms and decrease exacerbations.
      2. Therefore, consider in patients with moderate-to-severe
          airflow limitation and symptoms.
    iii. Combined β_2-agonists and inhaled corticosteroids
      1. Fluticasone/salmeterol (Advair Diskus) [100, 250, 500]/
          50 μg inhaled q12h
    iv. Theophylline (see Chapter 2.9)—may improve lung function
         and symptoms when added
  c. Supplemental therapy
    i. Oxygen—supplemental oxygen for those with saturation
        ≤88% (therefore Pao_2 ≤55 mm Hg)
    ii. Pulmonary rehabilitation
    iii. Surgery—lung-volume reduction surgery or lung transplant
IV. Psychiatric pearls, pointers, and parallels (see Chapter 2.9)

2.15

THE COMMON COLD

I. Evaluation
  a. General—the *common cold* is a lay term for mild upper respiratory
      illness.
  b. Clinical—self-limited disease restricted to the upper respiratory
      tract; mean duration is 7 to 10 days.
    i. Frequent symptoms—nasal discharge and congestion, sneez-
        ing, sore throat, and cough
    ii. Less frequent symptoms—hoarseness, headache, malaise,
         myalgia, lethargy, and fever

   c. Etiology—heterogeneous viral illness; common viral causes include:
      i. Rhinovirus (30%–50%)
      ii. Coronavirus (10%–15%)
      iii. Influenza virus (5%–15%)

NOTE:

Influenza is typically regarded as a distinct disease entity and separate from the common cold (see Chapter 2.40.)

---

      iv. Respiratory syncytial virus (RSV) (5%)
      v. Parainfluenza virus (5%)
      vi. Adenovirus (<5%)
      vii. Enterovirus (<5%)
      viii. Unknown (20%–30%)
   d. Epidemiology
      i. Incidence is inversely proportional to age.
      ii. Rate of infection increases rapidly in the fall and remains high in the winter (temperate zone).
   e. Risk factors—day care, psychologic stress, and so on
   f. Transmission
      i. Hand contact with secretions (often transmits infection)
      ii. Large-particle aerosols (transmits infection less often)
      iii. Small-particle aerosols
   g. Diagnosis—clinical; can use rapid antigen detection kits.
      i. Specimens of choice—nasopharyngeal aspirates and nasal wash specimens
   h. Complications—although usually self-limiting, bacterial complications such as the following may arise:
      i. Otitis media (the most common bacterial complication in children)
      ii. Sinusitis
      iii. Pneumonia
      iv. Asthma or chronic obstructive pulmonary disease (COPD) exacerbation

II. Treatment—targets symptoms; no antibiotics given viral etiology (unless complications suspected)
   a. Antitussives (control or prevent cough; indicated if cough is creating significant discomfort)
      i. Nonopioid
         1. Dextromethorphan (may be referred to as *DM*) 10 to 20 mg PO q4h
         2. Benzonatate (Tessalon Pearls) 100 to 200 mg PO TID
      ii. Opioid
         1. Codeine 10 to 20 mg PO q4h
   b. Expectorants (promote expulsion of phlegm)
      i. Guaifenesin 200 to 400 mg PO q4h
      ii. Guaifenesin SR (Mucinex) 600 mg q12h p.r.n.

    iii. For patients with diabetes mellitus, consider sugar-free, alcohol-free Diabetic Tussin EX (guaifenesin)

  c. Decongestants (decrease nasal congestion)
  i. Pseudoephedrine (Sudafed) 30 to 60 mg PO q6h p.r.n ($\times$ 1 week maximum)
  ii. Phenylephrine (Sudafed PE) 10 mg PO q4h p.r.n ($\times$ 1 week)
  iii. CAUTION—stimulates α_1-receptors $\rightarrow$ hypertension, arrhythmias, and so on

  d. First generation antihistamines (decrease sneezing and rhinorrhea; also sedating and decrease cognition)
  i. Diphenhydramine (Benadryl) 25 to 50 mg PO q4h p.r.n.
  ii. Chlorpheniramine 4 mg PO q4h p.r.n.

> **NOTE:**
>
> It is likely that the anticholinergic properties of first generation antihistamines help alleviate cough; moreover, second generation (nonsedating) antihistamines have little or no anticholinergic effect and fail to alleviate viral cough.

  e. Cough drops
  i. Menthol containing cough drops (Halls, Cepacol lozenges) PO q3h p.r.n.

  f. Pain relief and antipyretic
  i. Acetaminophen (Tylenol) 325 to 1,000 mg q6h PO p.r.n.

> **NOTE:**
>
> Many Tylenol products combine acetaminophen with an antitussive, expectorant, decongestant, and/or antihistamine.

  g. Antitussive/expectorant combination
  i. DM/guaifenesin (Robitussin DM) 10/100—take 10 mL PO q4h p.r.n.
  ii. Codeine/guaifenesin (Robitussin AC) 10/300 PO q4h
  iii. For diabetes mellitus patients, consider sugar free, alcohol free
    1. Diabetic Tussin DM (guaifenesin/dextromethorphan) 100/10—take 10 mL PO q4h p.r.n.

  h. Decongestant/expectorant combination (limit pseudoephedrine and phenylephrine products to 1-week use)
  i. Pseudoephedrine/guaifenesin (Guaifenex PSE 120) 120/600 mg PO q12h
  ii. Pseudoephedrine/guaifenesin (Anatuss LA) 120/400 mg PO q12h
  iii. Phenylephrine/guaifenesin (Entex LA) 30/400 mg PO q12h

  i. Decongestant/antihistamine combination (limit pseudoephedrine products to 1-week use)
  i. Pseudoephedrine/chlorpheniramine (Novafed A) 120/8 mg PO q12h

CONGESTIVE HEART FAILURE

I. Evaluation
   a. General—clinical syndrome which affects heart function; that is, the ability to fill and/or pump blood
   b. Clinical—dyspnea, fatigue, edema (lungs and legs); + jugular venous pressure (JVP), gallop (S_3), and crackles
   c. Laboratory findings—increase in brain natriuretic peptide (BNP)

NOTE:

Approximately 20% to 50% of those with heart failure have preserved systolic function (normal ejection fraction); hence, cardiac contraction is normal, but relaxation (~diastole) is abnormal.

---

   d. Classification
      i. New York Heart Association (NYHA) Functional Classification of Heart Failure (see Table 2.16.1)
      ii. American College of Cardiology/American Heart Association Stages of Heart Failure (see Table 2.16.2)
II. Common heart failure medications
   a. ACE-inhibitors—improve survival, decrease rate of hospitalization, decrease symptoms, and reverse remodeling.
      i. Lisinopril (Zestril, Prinivil) 5 to 40 mg PO daily
      ii. Enalapril (Vasotec) 2.5 to 20 mg PO BID
      iii. CAUTION—watch for hyperkalemia, angioedema, and cough
   b. Angiotensin-receptor blockers (ARBs)—to be used only in those who cannot tolerate ACE-inhibitors.

TABLE 2.16.1 New York Heart Association (NYHA) Functional Classification of Heart Failure

Class	Conditions
I	No symptoms with ordinary physical activity
II	Symptoms occur with ordinary physical activity; therefore, *mild* limitation of activity
III	Symptoms occur with less-than-ordinary physical activity; therefore, *marked* limitation of activity
IV	Symptoms occur at rest; therefore, *severe* limitation of activity

Adapted from Silver MA. *Heart failure. Rakel: Conn's current therapy 2006*, 58th ed. WB Saunders; 2006:409–414.

TABLE 2.16.2 American College of Cardiology/American Heart Association Stages of Heart Failure

	Patient Description	Potential Treatments
Stage A	Normal heart structure and function NO signs/symptoms Risk factors for CHF are apparent (i.e., HTN, CAD, ↑ cholesterol, DM, etc.)	1. Treat risk factors (HTN, CAD, ↑ cholesterol, DM, etc.) 2. Smoking cessation and weight loss 3. ACE-inhibitor/ARB as appropriate
Stage B	Abnormal heart structure and function NO signs/symptoms	1. Same as for stage A and 2. ACE-inhibitor/ARB in all patients 3. β-Blockers in select patients
Stage C[a]	Abnormal heart structure and function Symptoms of heart failure	1. Same as for stage A and 2. ACE-inhibitor/ARB in all patients 3. β-Blockers in all patients 4. Dietary sodium restriction/fluid restriction 5. Diuretics and digoxin in most patients 6. Cardiac resynchronization if bundle-branch block (e.g., biventricular pacemaker system) 7. Revascularization, repair mitral regurgitation (if present) 8. Aldosterone antagonist (e.g., Spironolactone), nesiritide
Stage D	- Extremely abnormal heart structure and function - Severe symptoms of heart failure	1. Same as for stage C and 2. Inotropes 3. Left ventricular assist device (LVAD) 4. Heart transplant 5. Hospice

[a] This is the stage where NYHA Functional Classification of Heart Failure becomes appropriate because symptoms are apparent in this stage.
CHF, congestive heart failure; HTN, hypertension; CAD, coronary artery disease; DM, diabetes mellitus; ACE, angiotensin-converting enzyme; ARB, angiotensin receptor blocker; NYHA, New York Heart Association.
(Adapted from Silver MA. *Heart failure. Rakel: Conn's current therapy 2006*, 58th ed. WB Saunders; 2006:409–414.)

    i.   Candesartan (Atacand) 4 to 32 mg PO daily
    ii. Valsartan (Diovan) 40 to 160 mg PO BID
    iii. CAUTION—watch for hyperkalemia and angioedema
  c. β-Blockers—counteracts harmful effects of sympathetic nervous system, improve survival, and decreases remodeling.
    i.   Metoprolol XL (Toprol XL) 12.5 to 200 mg PO daily (selective β₁-blocker)

        ii. Carvedilol (Coreg) 3.125 to 25 mg PO BID (nonselective β-blocker and selective α_1-blocker)

        iii. CAUTION—do not use immediately in patients with recent heart failure exacerbation

    d. Loop diuretics—used to control symptoms of congestion.

        i. Furosemide (Lasix) 40 to 120 mg PO daily to BID—doses may even get higher

        ii. CAUTION—hypokalemia; ototoxicity at higher doses

    e. Digoxin—no mortality benefit, but decrease worsening heart failure and hospitalization

        i. Digoxin (Lanoxin) 0.125 to 0.5 mg PO daily

        ii. CAUTION—adjustment needed for renal function; beware of toxicity (gastrointestinal [GI], neurologic, cardiac, and visual) (see Chapter 2.8)

    f. Aldosterone antagonists—decrease sodium retention, perhaps decrease organ fibrosis

        i. Spironolactone (Aldactone) 25 to 50 mg PO daily

        ii. CAUTION—hyperkalemia → sudden death!

III. Psychiatric pearls, pointers, and parallels

    a. β-Blockers are particularly important in psychiatry:

        i. Overdose with β-blockers leads to cardiotoxicity, bradycardia, and hypotension.

           1. Treatment

              a. Atropine 0.5 to 2 mg IM/IV STAT

              b. Glucagon 5 to 10 mg IM/IV STAT, followed by an infusion of 1 to 5 mg per hour

        ii. Depression and β-blockers

           1. Controversy surrounds this issue; therefore, it is unclear if β-blockers trigger/worsen depression.

              a. Central nervous system (CNS) effects are most common with those β-blockers that have greater lipid solubility.

                  i. Greater lipid solubility allows for easier crossing of the blood–brain barrier.

              b. Atenolol (Tenormin) has greater aqueous solubility and thereby less CNS effects.

CONJUNCTIVITIS (ACUTE)

I. Evaluation
   a. General—inflammation of the mucous membrane that covers the anterior surface of the eye from the inner surface of the eyelid to the corneal edge
   b. Clinical (in general)—"red/pink eye," "injected" blood vessels on eye's surface
   c. Etiology—infectious (viral, bacterial) or noninfectious (allergic, chemical)

REMEMBER:

In general, avoid prescribing topical steroids for acute conjunctivitis as they can cause multiple complications (including loss of sight); defer to an ophthalmologist.

II. Viral conjunctivitis ("pink eye")
   a. Clinical—(symptoms may persist for 2–3 weeks.)
      i. Acute redness (conjunctival injection), watery discharge, feels like foreign body irritation.
      ii. May have tender, enlarged preauricular lymph node.
      iii. If there are corneal infiltrates (small white dots on surface of cornea)—get ophthalmology consult.
   b. Transmission—secretions, fomites (e.g., towels), pools; usually bilateral from self-inoculation.
   c. Etiology—adenovirus is the most likely cause.
   d. Treatment
      i. Supportive—cool compresses, decrease lid edema, acetaminophen p.r.n.
      ii. Symptomatic relief from topical antihistamine/decongestant
         1. Naphazoline/pheniramine (Naphcon A) 1 to 2 drops OS/OD daily to QID p.r.n.
      iii. Keep hands and towels clean; avoid health care setting work for approximately 4 days
III. Bacterial conjunctivitis
   a. Clinical—acute/subacute redness, irritation, and purulent discharge with mattering at eyelid margin
   b. Transmission—direct contact
   c. Etiology—*Streptococcus* and *Staphylococcus* the two most common in adults
   d. Treatment, many choices—(Note: ointments provide better symptom relief, but can blur vision)
      i. Erythromycin ophthalmic 0.5% ointment—apply OS/OD up to q4h × 7 days

75

      ii. Bacitracin ophthalmic ointment—apply OS/OD q3h–q4h ×
         7 days

      iii. Polymyxin B/trimethoprim (Polytrim) 1 drop OS/OD q4h
         × 7 days

      iv. Sulfacetamide ophthalmic 10% solution (Bleph-10) 1 to 2
         drops OS/OD q2h to q3h × 7 days

      v. Ciprofloxacin ophthalmic (Ciloxan) 1 to 2 drops OS/OD
         q2h × 2 days, then q4h × 5 days

         1. Use fluoroquinolones against pseudomonas, that is, in
           contact lens conjunctivitis

IV. Gonococcal conjunctivitis

  a. Clinical

    i. Hyperacute red, irritated eye with copious purulent discharge
      and lid edema

    ii. Preauricular lymph node enlargement

    iii. Can cause corneal perforation, and therefore an ophthalmo-
      logic emergency

  b. Etiology—*Neisseria gonorrhoeae* (from genitourinary infection)

  c. Treatment—This is a medical emergency. Get ophthalmology
    consultation STAT!

    i. Ceftriaxone (Rocephin) 1 g IV q12h to q24h and topical
      ciprofloxacin q2h (at least)

    ii. Frequent eye irrigation

V. Chlamydial conjunctivitis

  a. Clinical—intermittent conjunctival injection, mucopurulent dis-
    charge

  b. Etiology—*Chlamydia trachomatis* (most often in young adults with
    concomitant genital infection)

  c. Transmission—hand-to-eye contact

  d. Treatment

    i. Azithromycin (Zithromax) 1 g × 1 dose

VI. Allergic conjunctivitis

  a. Description—an allergen causes a hypersensitivity reaction
    resulting in immunoglobulin E (IgE) and histamine release.

  b. Clinical—redness, pruritis, watery discharge; associated with sea-
    sonal allergies.

  c. Treatment—may use oral antihistamines (see Chapter 2.2)
    and

    i. Olopatadine ophthalmic (Patanol) 0.1% solution 1 to 2 drops
      OS/OD BID

    ii. Ketotifen ophthalmic (Zaditor) 0.025% solution 1 drop
      OS/OD BID

REMEMBER:

Pain, decreased vision, or cloudy cornea are not usually found with conjunctivitis. These factors should alert one to a more serious problem; consult
ophthalmology.

CONSTIPATION (CHRONIC)

I. Evaluation
   a. General—Rome II diagnostic criteria necessitates two or more of the following for ≥12 weeks in the past year:
      i. Straining during >25% of bowel movements (BMs)
      ii. Hard stools for >25% of BMs
      iii. Sensation of incomplete evacuation for >25% of BMs
      iv. Sensation of anorectal blockage for >25% of BMs
      v. Manual maneuvers to assist with >25% of BMs
      vi. Less than three BMs per week (for severe constipation, BMs only twice a month)
   b. Epidemiology—3♀: 1♂; nonwhites > whites; elderly > young adults
   c. Risk factors—inactivity, low income, limited education, sexual abuse history, and major depression
   d. Classification
      i. Normal-transit constipation—most common type
         1. Clinical
            a. BMs have a normal frequency, yet patients perceive being constipated.
            b. Usually have hard stools, bloating, and abdominal discomfort.
         2. Treatment—use dietary fiber. May add an osmotic laxative if needed.
      ii. Defecatory disorders (anismus)
         1. Clinical
            a. It is usually due to pelvic floor or anal sphincter dysfunction.
            b. May result from resisting urge to defecate, structural abnormality, and so on.
            c. Some patients have a history of abuse or an eating disorder.
      iii. Slow-transit constipation
         1. Clinical—often starts at puberty and seen in ♀ who have infrequent BMs (<1/week).
         2. Pathology—some studies have shown alteration in myenteric plexus neurons.
         3. Treatment—dietary fiber.
II. Differential diagnosis
   a. Primary constipation
      i. Functional (irritable bowel syndrome [IBS], anismus, slow-transit constipation, etc.)

     ii. Structural—obstructive (Crohn's disease, colon cancer, stricture, etc.)

     iii. Gynecologic (pelvic relaxation, large rectocele, etc.)

     iv. Neuropathic (Hirschsprung's disease, spinal cord injury, etc.)

   b. Secondary constipation

     i. Endocrine and metabolic (diabetes mellitus, hypothyroidism, hypercalcemia, pregnancy, etc.)

     ii. Lifestyle (low fiber, dehydration, sedentary, etc.)

     iii. Smooth muscle and connective tissue (amyloidosis, scleroderma, etc.)

     iv. Medications (anticholinergics, antidepressants, antipsychotics, iron, opiates, etc.)

     v. Psychogenic (depression, stress, somatization, anxiety, eating disorders, etc.)

     vi. Neuropathic (Parkinson's disease, multiple sclerosis, autonomic neuropathy, etc.)

III. Treatment

   a. Nonpharmacologic

     i. Healthy lifestyle (increase fluid intake, increase fiber, increase physical activity)

       1. Few data support that patients get constipation relief with changes in lifestyle.

       2. Limit caffeine and alcohol as they increase renal elimination of fluids and decrease gastrointestinal (GI) elimination.

     ii. Disimpaction—manually remove fecal impaction

     iii. Biofeedback—good for defecatory disorders

     iv. Acupuncture

     v. Surgery—last resort for refractory constipation

   b. Pharmacologic

     i. Bulk laxatives take with plenty of water; titrate slowly to avoid flatulence, bloating, and so on.

       1. Psyllium (Metamucil, Fiberall)—titrate over 1 to 2 weeks to 20 g per day

       2. Methylcellulose (Citrucel)—titrate over 1to 2 weeks to 20 g per day

       3. Polycarbophil (Fibercon)—titrate over 1 to 2 weeks to 20 g per day

     ii. Osmotic laxatives—poorly absorbed; take days to work; secrete water into intestines.

       1. Magnesium hydroxide (Milk of Magnesia) 15 to 30 mL PO daily to BID

       2. Magnesium citrate (Evac-Q-Mag) 150 to 300 mL PO p.r.n.

       3. Sodium phosphate (Fleet Phospho-Soda) 10 to 25 mL PO with water p.r.n.

       4. CAUTION—avoid in patients with renal insufficiency or cardiac dysfunction

   iii. Poorly absorbed sugars
       1. Lactulose 15 to 30 mL PO daily to BID
       2. Polyethylene glycol and electrolytes (Colyte, GoLYTELY) 17 to 36 g PO daily to BID
       3. Polyethylene glycol 3,350 (Miralax) 17 to 36 g PO daily to BID
           a. Miralax may take 2 to 4 days to produce a bowel movement.
   iv. Stimulant laxatives—increase intestinal motility and secretions; work within hours.
       1. Anthraquinones
           a. Senna (Senokot, Ex-Lax) one to two tablets PO daily to BID
       2. Diphenylmethane derivatives
           a. Bisacodyl (Dulcolax) 5 to 10 mg PO qhs
       3. Stool softener—allows water to interact more effectively with stool
           a. Docusate sodium (Colace) 100 mg PO BID
           b. Docusate calcium (Surfak) 240 mg PO BID
       4. Castor oil (Emulsoil) 15 to 30 mL PO daily
       5. Mineral oil (Fleet mineral oil) 5 to 15 mL PO qhs
   v. Rectal enema/suppository—distends rectum, softens stool, stimulates muscle contraction.
       1. Tap-water enema 500 mL daily
       2. Soapsuds enema 1,500 mL daily
       3. Milk of molasses enema
       4. Phosphate enema (Fleet enema) 120 mL daily
       5. CAUTION—electrolyte abnormalities can occur if the enema is retained
   vi. Cholinergic agent—appears beneficial in those with constipation from tricyclic antidepressants (TCAs).
       1. Bethanechol (Urecholine) 10 mg PO daily (also helps with TCA-associated bladder dysfunction)
   vii. Prokinetic agent (5-HT$_4$-receptor agonist)—decreases pain and bloating, increases BM frequency.
       1. Tegaserod (Zelnorm) 6 mg PO BID × 4 to 6 weeks
           a. Used in patients with IBS.
IV. Psychiatric pearls, pointers, and parallels
   a. Psychiatric medications (typically due to anticholinergic side effects) are often implicated in constipation.
   b. Constipation can also be a symptom of somatoform disorders.

COUGH

I. Differential diagnosis of acute cough (cough lasting <3 weeks)
   a. Common cold (see Chapter 2.15)
   b. Allergic rhinitis (see Chapter 2.2)
   c. Acute bacterial sinusitis (see Chapter 2.48)
   d. Chronic obstructive pulmonary disease (COPD) exacerbation (see Chapter 2.14).
   e. Bordetella pertussis infection
      i. Treatment—erythromycin 500 mg QID OR Trimethoprim-sulfamethoxazole (TMP-SMZ) 160/800 mg BID × 14 days

> **REMEMBER:**
>
> Acute cough can be the presenting symptom of pneumonia, heart failure, asthma, and so on.

II. Differential diagnosis of subacute cough (cough lasting 3–8 weeks)
   a. Respiratory infection → treat! (see Chapter 2.47)
   b. Postinfectious cough—begins with an acute respiratory tract infection and no evidence of pneumonia
      i. Antihistamine (e.g., diphenhydramine) + decongestant (e.g., pseudoephedrine) × 1 week
      Ipratropium (Atrovent) metered dose inhaler (MDI)—four puffs QID for 1 to 3 weeks
      ii. If no response to the above dosage, then prednisone 40 mg per day × 3 days and taper over 2 to 3 weeks.
   c. Subacute bacterial sinusitis (see Chapter 2.48)
   d. Asthma (see Chapter 2.9)
   e. Bordetella pertussis infection
      i. Treatment—erythromycin 500 mg QID OR TMP-SMZ 160/800 mg BID × 14 days
III. Differential diagnosis of chronic cough (cough lasting >8 weeks)
   a. Ninety-five percent of cases for immunocompetent patients include
      i. Postnasal-drip syndromes
         1. Nonallergic rhinitis
            a. Antihistamine + decongestant × 3 weeks
            OR ipratropium 0.06% nasal spray (Atrovent nasal) BID × 3 weeks
         2. Allergic rhinitis (see Chapter 2.2)
         3. Vasomotor rhinitis

a. Ipratropium 0.06% nasal spray BID × 3 weeks and thereafter p.r.n.
   4. Chronic bacterial sinusitis (see Chapter 2.48)
ii. Asthma (see Chapter 2.9).
iii. Gastroesophageal reflux disease (GERD) (see Chapter 2.29)
iv. Chronic bronchitis (due to cigarette smoking or another irritant)
   1. Eliminate the irritant (i.e., stop smoking)
   2. Ipratropium (Atrovent) MDI two puffs QID
v. Eosinophilic bronchitis
   1. Budesonide inhaled (Pulmicort Turbuhaler) two puffs (400 μg) BID × 2 weeks.
   2. If no response, prednisone 30 mg per day for 2 to 3 weeks (may need long-term treatment).
vi. Angiotensin-converting enzyme (ACE)-inhibitor use
   1. Discontinue ACE-inhibitor as cough is NOT dose-related; consider angiotensin-receptor blocker.
   2. Cough should improve within 4 weeks.
b. Five percent of cases for immunocompetent patients include
   i. Left ventricular failure—congestive heart failure
   ii. Carcinomatosis
   iii. Carcinoma/malignancy
   iv. Aspiration
   v. Sarcoidosis

REMEMBER:

Many times chronic cough has more than one cause.

2.20

DENTAL PROCEDURES PROPHYLAXIS IN PATIENTS AT RISK

I. Evaluation
   a. General—dental work causes transient bacteremia that may result in endocarditis in at-risk patients.
   b. Etiology—the most common cause of endocarditis postdental procedure is *Streptococcus viridans*.

   c. Cardiac conditions associated with endocarditis
      i. High/moderate risk
         1. Prosthetic heart valve
         2. Acquired heart valve dysfunction (e.g., because of rheumatic heart disease)
         3. Mitral valve prolapse with mitral regurgitation and/or thickened leaflets
         4. Previous history of bacterial endocarditis
         5. Surgically made pulmonary shunts or conduits
         6. Congenital heart disease (e.g., tetralogy of Fallot, etc.)
         7. Hypertrophic cardiomyopathy
   d. Dental procedures for which antibiotic prophylaxis is recommended in at-risk patients.
      i. Periodontal procedures
      ii. Dental extractions
      iii. Dental implant placement
      iv. Dental cleaning of teeth or implants where bleeding is expected
      v. Endodontic instrumentation (root canal)
      vi. Intraligamentary local anesthetic injections
      vii. Placement of orthodontic bands
      viii. Subgingival placement of antibiotic fibers/strips
   e. Prophylactic regimens (see Table 2.20.1)

TABLE **2.20.1** Prophylactic Regimens	
Standard	Amoxicillin 2 g PO 1 hr before procedure
Unable to take PO	Ampicillin 2 g IM/IV 30-min before procedure
Penicillin allergy	Clindamycin (Cleocin) 600 mg PO 1 hr before procedure
	or clindamycin (Cleocin) 600 mg IV 30-min before procedure
	OR
	Azithromycin (Zithromax) 500 mg PO 1 hr before procedure
	or clarithromycin (Biaxin) 500 mg PO 1 hr before procedure
	OR
	Cephalexin* (Keflex) 2 g PO 1 hr before procedure
	or Cefazolin* (Ancef) 1 g IV 30 min before procedure

Adapted from Dajani AS, Taubert KA, Wilson W, et al. Prevention of bacterial endocarditis: Recommendations by the American Heart Association. *Clin Infect Dis.* 1997;25:1448–1458.

---

*REMEMBER:

Up to 10% of patients with a penicillin allergy have an adverse reaction to cephalosporins. Those who claim severe or anaphylactic reaction to penicillin should avoid cephalosporins. If needed, an allergy consult is recommended.

DIABETES MELLITUS

I. Evaluation
   a. General—includes many diseases of abnormal carbohydrate metabolism with resultant hyperglycemia
   b. Diagnostic criteria (use any of the following, but results *must be confirmed* on a separate day)
      i. Nonfasting blood sugar (BS) >200 mg per dL = diabetes mellitus (DM)
      ii. Fasting blood sugar (FBS) or fasting plasma glucose (FPG)
         1. Normal = <100 mg per dL
         2. Impaired fasting glucose (IFG) ("prediabetes") = 100 to 125 mg per dL
         3. DM = >126 mg per dL
      iii. Oral glucose tolerance test (OGTT)—give 75 g of PO glucose, then 2 hours later, obtain BS
         1. Normal = <140 mg per dL
         2. Impaired glucose tolerance (IGT) ("prediabetes") = 140 to 199 mg per dL
         3. DM = >200 mg per dL

NOTE:

HbA$_{1c}$ (glycosylated hemoglobin) is currently NOT recommended for the diagnosis of DM.

---

   c. Clinical—polyphagia, polydipsia, polyuria, nocturia, weight loss, fatigue, and blurred vision
   d. Epidemiology—approximately 25 million Americans have DM (diagnosed and undiagnosed combined)
II. DM type I (formerly insulin-dependent DM)
   a. Pathology—pancreatic β-cell destruction (through autoimmune attack or idiopathic) results in a decrease in insulin.
   b. Epidemiology—5% to 10% of all cases of DM; occurs at low incidence level throughout adulthood.
   c. Risk factors
      i. Family history (particularly, a first-degree relative with DM type I)
         1. Susceptibility predominantly rests with human leucocyte antigen (HLA) genotypes DR and DQ
      ii. Race (white, particularly those from northern Europe)
   d. Management theory
      i. Concepts as gleaned from the Diabetes Control and Complications Trial (DCCT)

1. Any decrease in HbA_{1c} is associated with a decrease in relative risk of complications (microvascular [retinopathy, nephropathy, and neuropathy] and likely macrovascular).
2. Intensive management should be implemented once DM is diagnosed.
3. Hypoglycemia ($\rightarrow$ cognitive impairment) is a limiting step in managing DM.

e. Management components
   i. Insulin
      1. Types (see Table 2.21.1)

NOTE:

Humulin 70/30 is a premixed insulin with 70% NPH and 30% regular insulin.

---

   2. Basal-bolus insulin therapy approach uses multiple daily injections or an insulin pump.
      a. "Basal" supply of insulin allows the presence of a low level of insulin through the day, and is provided by intermediate, long, or very long-acting preparations given qhs or BID.
      b. "Bolus" supply of insulin is needed to cover the expected rise in blood glucose after a meal, and is provided by the rapid or fast-acting preparations, given before meals and based on carbohydrate counting in grams or as determined by a sliding scale.
         i. Sliding scale formula—for BS >150 mg per dL
            1. Give ($[BS - 150]/25$) units of regular insulin SC
   3. Determining insulin dosage by the Rule of Thirds (when dosage is unknown)

TABLE 2.21.1 Types of Insulin				
Insulin	**Type**	**Onset**	**Peak**	**Duration**
Lispro (Humalog)	Rapid acting	5–10 min	30 min–2 hr	3–4 hr
Regular (Humulin R/Novolin R)	Fast acting	30 min–1 hr	2–5 hr	6–8 hr
NPH (Humulin N/Novolin N)	Intermediate	1–2 hr	4–14 hr	16–26 hr
Ultralente (Humulin U)	Long acting	3–4 hr	8–15 hr	22–26 hr
Glargine (Lantus)	Very long	30 min–1 hr	—	20–24 hr

(Adapted from Daneman D. Type 1 diabetes. *Lancet.* 2006;367:847–858, with additional information from Micromedex, http://www.micromedex.com.)

       a. Total daily insulin requirement = 0.5 to 1.2 units/kg/day.

       b. Give two thirds of insulin as intermediate acting, one third as short acting.

       c. Give two thirds of intermediate insulin before the AM meal, one third before the PM meal.

       d. Adjust based on blood glucose monitoring results—monitor qAC and qhs.

          i. PM BS reflects adequacy of AM insulin dose.

          ii. AM BS reflects adequacy of prior PM's insulin dose.

  ii. Nutritional planning

    1. Tailor to the needs/preferences of the patient to improve compliance.

    2. Consistency in meal planning can help in obtaining glycemic targets.

    3. Complex carbohydrates and monounsaturated fat should only be 60% to 70% of energy intake.

  iii. Microvascular complications of DM type I

    1. Diabetic nephropathy

      a. Epidemiology—most common cause of renal failure in the developed world

      b. Phases

        i. Microalbuminuria—urinary albumin excretion 20 to 200 μg per day

        ii. Macroalbuminura—urinary albumin excretion >200 μg per day

        iii. End-stage renal disease

      c. Screening—annual urine albumin–creatinine ratio in patients with diabetes ≥5 years

      d. Treatment—improve glycemic, blood pressure, and lipid control; angiotensin-converting enzyme inhibitor (ACE)-I or angiotensin receptor blocker (ARB)

    2. Diabetic retinopathy

      a. Epidemiology—most common cause of acquired blindness in the developed world

      b. Phases

        i. Early nonproliferative changes (microaneurysms, exudates)

        ii. Preproliferative retinopathy

        iii. Proliferative retinopathy (risk of retinal detachment, etc.)

      c. Screening—annual fundus examination in patients with diabetes ≥5 years

      d. Treatment—improve glycemic, blood pressure, and lipid control; laser therapy

    3. Diabetic neuropathy

      a. Focal, generalized, or autonomic

      b. Peripheral neuropathy + peripheral vascular disease (PVD) → skin ulceration → diabetic foot

         i. Therefore, a foot examination is important annually in patients with diabetes ≥5 years.

      c. Treatment—improve glycemic control

    iv. Macrovascular complications of diabetes mellitus type I

      1. Cardiovascular

REMEMBER:

DM is a coronary artery disease risk equivalent.

---

        a. Treatment—improve glycemic control and reduce risk of vascular disease (smoking cessation, blood pressure <130/80, low-density lipoprotein [LDL] <100, exercise, control weight).

      2. Cerebrovascular

      3. Peripheral vascular disease

III. DM type II (formerly noninsulin-dependent DM)

  a. Pathology—begins with insulin insensitivity as pancreas β-cell function declines over time.

  b. Epidemiology—approximately 90% of all cases of DM.

  c. Risk factors

    i. Age older than 45 years

    ii. Obesity (body mass index [BMI] >30)

    iii. Lack of physical activity (exercise <3 times/week)

    iv. Family history (particularly, a first-degree relative with DM type II)

    v. High-risk ethnic group (African American, Hispanic, Native American, Asian and Pacific Islander)

    vi. Delivery of a baby >9 lb and/or gestational diabetes

    vii. Hypertension (≥140/90)

    viii. Dyslipidemia (high-density lipoprotein [HDL] <35 mg dL, triglycerides [TG] >250 mg/dL)

    ix. Impaired fasting glucose (IFG) or impaired glucose tolerance (IGT)

  d. Oral agents for treatment—(each of these medications can lower HbA_{1c} by ~1%–1.5%)

    i. Thiazolidinediones

      1. Mechanism of action—enhance insulin sensitivity; ameliorate dyslipidemia

      2. Adverse effects

        a. Fluid retention (worsens congestive heart failure [CHF]), increase in weight

        b. Monitor for liver toxicity by following liver function tests (LFTs) every 2 months

      3. Medications

        a. Pioglitazone (Actos) 15 to 45 mg PO daily

  b. Rosiglitazone (Avandia) 4 to 8 mg PO daily or divided BID
 ii. Biguanides
   1. Mechanism of action—decrease hepatic glucose output
   2. Adverse effects—gastrointestinal (GI) symptoms, lactic acidosis

---

REMEMBER:

Although rare, lactic acidosis (nonspecific symptoms include hyperventilation, dyspnea, severe weakness, myalgia, abdominal distress, drowsiness) can be fatal; therefore, do NOT use metformin in those with ↓ glomerular filtration rate (GFR), CHF, alcoholism, or abnormal liver function.

---

   3. Medications
     a. Metformin (Glucophage) 850 mg PO daily, titrate up to 2,550 mg per day (divided BID)
     b. Metformin XR (Glucophage XR) 500 to 2,000 mg PO every evening
 iii. Second generation sulfonylurea derivatives (secretagogues)
   1. Mechanism of action—enhance insulin secretion
   2. Adverse effects
     a. Hypoglycemia (especially long-acting formulations), increase in weight
     b. Use with caution in the presence of liver or kidney impairment
   3. Medications
     a. Glipizide (Glucotrol) 2.5 to 20 mg PO daily (short acting)
     b. Glyburide (DiaBeta, Micronase) 1.25 to 20 mg PO daily (long acting)
 iv. α-Glucosidase inhibitors
   1. Mechanism of action—delay GI absorption of carbohydrates
   2. Adverse effects—GI symptoms common (flatulence, discomfort), increase in weight
   3. Medications
     a. Acarbose (Precose) 25 to 100 mg TID at the start of each meal
 e. Additional treatments
   i. Exogenous insulin (see Section II)
     1. General—the natural history is oral agent failure as β-cell function declines.
     2. Step-wise therapy
       a. Add an intermediate or long-acting insulin at bedtime to oral agents.
         i. NPH .15 to .2 units per kg at bedtime
         ii. Glargine .15 units per kg at bedtime

        b. If bedtime insulin + oral agents is not enough, stop sulfonylureas and begin an insulin regimen as outlined in the preceding text (see Section II).

   ii. Diet and exercise—weight loss through hypocaloric diets is key

      1. General—can decrease insulin resistance and decrease HbA$_{1c}$ by 0.5% to 2.0%.

  f. New treatments

   i. Exenatide (Byetta) 5 to 10 μg SC BID 1 hour before meals

      1. Mechanism of action—increase insulin secretion; an incretin mimetic

   ii. Inhaled insulin (Exubera).05 mg per kg inhaled TID

      1. Adverse effects—bronchospasm (rare), respiratory disorders, and hypoglycemia

  g. Management guidelines

   i. HbA$_{1c}$ <7%—monitor every 3 to 6 months to assess diabetes control

   ii. Blood pressure <130/80 (consider ACE-I; Heart Outcomes Prevention Evaluation [HOPE] study and benefit of ramipril)

   iii. LDL <100, HDL >45, TG <200 (consider statin; 4 S Study and Heart Protection Study)

   iv. Aspirin 81 mg daily as prevention against consequences of atherosclerotic disease

  h. Microvascular and macrovascular complications of DM type II (see Section II).

IV. Potentially life-threatening acute complications of diabetes mellitus

  a. Hypoglycemia

   i. Definition—plasma glucose <50 mg per dL

   ii. Clinical

      1. Adrenergic—sweating, tremors, anxiety, increased heart rate, and palpitations

      2. Neuroglycopenic—visual disturbances, behavioral changes, seizures, and coma

   iii. Treatment

      1. For conscious patient—three glucose tablets, or half cup of juice

        a. Repeat BS; if low, repeat the above treatment

      2. For unconscious patient—25 to 50 g of 50% dextrose IV OR (if no IV access), Glucagon 0.5 to 1 mg IM/SC

        a. Glucagon may cause vomiting, so take precautions to prevent aspiration.

        b. It is short acting, so hypoglycemia may recur if no PO glucose is given.

> **NOTE:**
>
> Any patient with fasting hypoglycemia of unexplained etiology needs to be assessed for *factitious hypoglycemia*; check plasma insulin, C-peptide (normal/decreased with exogenous insulin), and/or urine sulfonylurea levels (rule out overdose).

   b. Diabetic ketoacidosis (DKA)
      i. Definition—due to severe insulin deficiency; therefore, glucose does not go to cells for energy
      ii. Clinical
         1. Symptoms—nausea, emesis, polyuria, polydipsia, abdominal pain, stupor, and coma
         2. Physical—dehydrated, altered mental status, air hunger (Kussmaul), and fruity breath
      iii. Etiology—usually precipitated by infectious process, poor compliance, or medical illness
      iv. Laboratory findings—glucose >300, pH <7.3, Pco_2 <40, HCO_3 <15, increased anion gap (AG), ketones in serum/urine
      v. Treatment—best treated in the intensive care unit (ICU); need significant fluid replacement, insulin, and potassium
         1. Of course, rule out precipitating factors.
   c. Nonketotic hyperosmolar syndrome
      i. Definition—extreme hyperglycemia and serum hyperosmolarity without ketoacidosis
      ii. Clinical
         1. Symptoms—nausea, emesis, polyuria, delirium, seizures, and coma (25% of patients)
         2. Physical—extremely dehydrated, neuro deficits, orthostatic, and tachycardia
      iii. Etiology—precipitated by severe dehydration, infection, stress, missed medicines, or new-onset diabetes
      iv. Laboratory findings—glucose >600 mg per dL, serum osmolarity >310, blood urea nitrogen (BUN) approximately 60 to 90, ketonemia is absent or mild
         1. Although serum electrolytes appear normal, tissue electrolytes may actually be low.
      v. Treatment—best treated in a medical center; need fluids, insulin, and typically potassium replacement
         1. Of course, rule out precipitating factors.
V. Psychiatric pearls, pointers, and parallels
   a. Patients on atypical antipsychotics should be informed of the potential risk for developing diabetes.

b. Depression and diabetes appear to be independent risk factors for white matter changes seen on magnetic resonance imaging (MRI).
c. The presence of diabetes increases the risk of comorbid affective disorders and psychotic disorders.
    i. Possible mechanisms of comorbidity
        1. Obesity
        2. Genetic components
        3. Alteration in cerebral glucose utilization
        4. Increased release of counterregulatory hormones as in the stress response

2.22

DIARRHEA

I. Diarrhea
    a. General—decrease in stool consistency, increase in stool frequency, urgency, ± abdominal discomfort
        i. Objective definition → stool weight >200 g per day (misses 20% of diarrheal symptoms)
    b. Etiology—usually due to changes in intestinal fluid and electrolyte transport
    c. Classification
        i. Acute—typically <2 to 3 weeks; rarely 6 to 8 weeks long; mostly self-limited
        ii. Chronic—lasts at least 4 weeks; usually >6 to 8 weeks long; unlikely self-limited
II. Acute diarrhea
    a. Diagnostic algorithm
        i. Delineate between infectious and noninfectious causes
            1. If infectious, assess severity, duration, setting, and host (i.e., is host immunocompetent?)
                a. Is acute diarrhea "medically important?" (≥1 present)
                    i. Severe dehydration
                    ii. Duration >3 days
                    iii. Fecal white blood corpuscles (WBCs) or bloody diarrhea
                        1. Nosocomial diarrhea? Traveler's diarrhea?
                    iv. Local outbreak (food-borne, etc.)

      v. Impaired host (acquired immunodeficiency syndrome [AIDS], etc.)

   b. If "medically important" obtain pertinent cultures, *Clostridium difficile* toxin, and so on

---

NOTE:

Approximately 20% to 40% of all acute infectious diarrheas remain undiagnosed.

---

  b. Management
     i. Fluid and electrolyte replacement—death in acute diarrhea is usually from dehydration
    ii. Symptomatic treatments
       1. Bismuth subsalicylate (Pepto-Bismol) two tablets (= 525 mg) PO q1h p.r.n. (maximum 4,200 mg/day)
         a. Safe in bacterial infectious diarrhea

REMEMBER:

Opiates and anticholinergic drugs are NOT recommended for infectious diarrhea because they may worsen microorganism colonization by paralyzing intestinal motility and prolonging their excretion.

---

         b. Loperamide (Imodium) 4 mg × 1, then 2 mg PO p.r.n. (maximum 16 mg/day)
           i. Note: Safe in traveler's diarrhea without dysentery
         c. Diphenoxylate/atropine (Lomotil) two tablets PO QID (maximum eight tablets/day)
  c. Differential diagnosis
     i. Infectious diarrhea
       1. Transmission—fecal-oral from water, food, or person-to-person
       2. Clinical—nausea, vomiting, abdominal pain + diarrhea
         a. Watery, malabsorptive, or bloody diarrhea and fever (dysentery)
       3. Etiology—common
         a. Bacterial—*Campylobacter, Salmonella, Shigella, C. difficile, Escherichia coli*
         b. Viral ("viral gastroenteritis")—Norwalk agent (calicivirus), rotavirus
       4. Antibiotics (for certain non–*C. difficile* diarrheas, i.e., shigellosis, traveler's, etc.)
         a. While awaiting stool cultures to guide therapy, empirically use
           i. Fluoroquinolones (e.g., Ciprofloxacin) OR trimethoprim-sulfamethoxazole (TMP-SMZ) (second-line therapy)

NOTE:

Antibiotics are NOT recommended in treating *E. coli* O157:H7 (enterohemorrhagic) because the incidence of complications (i.e., hemolytic uremic syndrome) can be greater after such therapy.

---

       5. Antibiotics (for *C. difficile* that causes diarrhea through A and B toxins)
         a. Metronidazole (Flagyl) 500 mg PO q8h × 10 to 14 days
       6. Prevention—hand washing, good hygiene
    ii. Food-borne poisonings, for example, monosodium glutamate (MSG)
    iii. Antibiotic-associated diarrhea (up to 20% of patients on broad-spectrum antibiotics)

III. Brief differential diagnosis of chronic diarrhea (have patient evaluated by a specialist)
  a. Fatty diarrhea (steatorrhea = excess fat in stool; oily, foul-smelling)
    i. Malabsorption syndromes (short bowel, postresection, mucosal diseases, celiac sprue)
      1. Those with malabsorption can also have vitamin and mineral deficiencies.
      2. Celiac sprue has neuropsychologic symptoms including ataxia, depression, and anxiety.
    ii. Maldigestion (pancreatic insufficiency, bile acid deficiency)
  b. Inflammatory diarrhea
    i. Inflammatory bowel disease
    ii. Infectious diseases
      1. Protracted infection may occur with *E. coli, Giardia, Cryptosporidium,* and so on.
      2. Tropical sprue (malabsorption of nutrients, especially folic acid and B_{12})
    iii. Ischemic colitis
    iv. Radiation colitis
    v. Neoplasia
  c. Watery diarrhea
    i. Osmotic (osmotic gap >125 mOsm/kg)
      1. Carbohydrate malabsorption
         a. Lactose intolerance (most common cause in this category)
      2. Magnesium, phosphate, sulfate ingestion (e.g., osmotic laxatives)
    ii. Secretory (10 to 20 bowel movements per day suggests secretory diarrhea; osmotic gap <50 mOsm/kg)
      1. Congenital syndromes
      2. Disordered motility (diabetic autonomic neuropathy, hyperthyroidism, irritable bowel, etc.)

  3. Drugs, poisons, and bacterial toxins
  4. Neuroendocrine tumors
  5. Nonosmotic laxatives (laxative abuse)
IV. Psychiatric pearls, pointers, and parallels
  a. Psychiatric medications are often implicated in diarrhea.
    i. For example, gastrointestinal side effects of selective sero-
      tonin reuptake inhibitors (SSRIs), toxic levels of lithium, and
      so on
  b. Diarrhea can also be a symptom of somatoform disorders.
  c. Irritable bowel syndrome (IBS) is common in patients with
    anxiety disorders.

2.23

DYSMENORRHEA (MENSTRUAL CRAMPS)

I. Evaluation
  a. General—crampy pelvic pain beginning just before or at the
    onset of menses and lasting 1 to 3 days
  b. Etiology—thought to be from prostaglandin release in menstrual
    fluid, which causes uterine contraction and pain
  c. Classification
    i. Primary—typically begins in the first 6 months after menar-
      che; normal pelvic anatomy
      1. Epidemiology—prevalence ranges widely from 20% to
        90%
      2. Risk factors
        a. Age 20 years or younger
        b. Nulliparity
        c. Heavy menses
        d. Smoking
        e. Weight loss attempts independent of body mass in-
          dex (BMI)
        f. Depression, anxiety, or disruption of social support
          network

NOTE:

Ideally, a pelvic examination should be performed in sexually active women
with dysmenorrhea to screen for sexually transmitted diseases (STDs).

3. Treatment
   a. Nonsteroidal anti-inflammatory drug (NSAIDS) (e.g., Ibuprofen 400–800 mg PO QID × 2–3 days)
      i. Mechanism of action—inhibit prostaglandin synthesis
   b. Cyclo-oxygenase-2 (COX-2) inhibitors (e.g., Celecoxib 200 mg PO BID × 2–3 days)
   c. Oral contraceptive pills (OCPs), or depo-medroxyprogesterone (Depo-Provera)
      i. Mechanism of action—decrease prostaglandin release
   d. Alternatives
      i. Continuous low-level topical heat
      ii. Low-fat vegetarian diet
      iii. Aerobic exercise
      iv. Physical remedies (e.g., acupuncture, spinal manipulation, etc.)
      v. Supplements (e.g., thiamine, vitamin E, omega-3, etc.)
      vi. Herbals (e.g., Toki-shakuyakusan [TSS], etc.)
   ii. Secondary—occurs after years of painless menstruation; due to pelvic organ pathology
      1. Differential diagnosis (have patient evaluated by a specialist)
         a. Endometriosis or adenomyosis
         b. Pelvic inflammation
         c. Uterine fibroids
         d. Ovarian cysts or tumor
         e. Pelvic anatomic abnormality

REMEMBER:

The onset of secondary dysmenorrhea demands a full abdominal and pelvic examination.

II. Psychiatric pearls, pointers, and parallels
   a. Pelvic pain is often labeled a "psychiatric problem" because
      i. It is often a clue to prior sexual or physical trauma.
      ii. It is often implicated in somatoform disorders.
   b. Have a gynecologist rule out organic causes of acute or chronic pelvic pain.

DYSPEPSIA

I. Evaluation
   a. General—"bad digestion" translated from Greek
   b. Clinical—varied symptoms → upper abdominal discomfort, early satiety, bloating, nausea, and emesis
   c. Etiology
      i. Forty percent organic—gastroduodenal ulcer (15%–25%), gastroesophageal reflux disease (GERD) (5%–15%), gastric cancer (<2%)
      ii. Sixty percent "functional" or idiopathic—nonulcer dyspepsia
         1. Rome II diagnostic criteria (criteria met for ≥12 weeks)
            a. Persistent or recurrent symptoms (as outlined earlier)
            b. An organic disease not found to explain the symptoms
            c. Diagnosis not better described as irritable bowel syndrome (IBS)
         2. Subclassification of nonulcer dyspepsia
            a. Ulcer-like ("burning" pain)
            b. Dysmotility-like (nausea, bloating or distension, early satiety)
            c. Unspecified
II. Differential diagnosis of nonulcer dyspepsia
   a. Nonmotility disorders
      i. Gastritis (possible *Helicobacter pylori* infection)
      ii. Duodenitis
      iii. Maldigestion/malabsorption of carbohydrates (e.g., lactose intolerance)
      iv. Small intestine parasite
      v. Pancreatitis
      vi. Psychiatric disorder
   b. Motility disorders
      i. Nonerosive esophageal reflux disease
      ii. Gastroparesis
      iii. Small intestine dysmotility
      iv. Biliary dysmotility
III. Diagnostic approach to dyspepsia
   a. Triage by history
      i. If serious risk factors (age 50 years or older, dysphagia, palpable mass, unexplained weight loss, protracted vomiting, or evidence of bleeding), then work up with endoscopy, and so on.
      ii. If *no* serious risk factors or above-mentioned workup is negative, then consider nonulcer dyspepsia.

1. Treat with a trial of antisecretory medications.
   a. Antacids—usually provide little help, especially for chronic dyspepsia
      i. Maalox (aluminum and magnesium hydroxide) 15 to 30 mL PO QID p.r.n.
      ii. Mylanta (Maalox + Simethicone) 15 to 30 mL PO QID p.r.n.
   b. Proton pump inhibitor (PPI)—50% of patients respond
      i. Omeprazole (Prilosec) 20 to 40 mg PO daily (see Chapter 2.29)
2. Consider additional treatments (symptom targeted).
   a. Prokinetic
      i. Metoclopramide (Reglan) 5 to 10 mg PO q6h
         1. Adverse effects Antidopaminergic
   b. Antiflatulent
      i. Simethicone (Mylicon) 80 to 120 mg PO QID p.r.n.
      ii. Mylanta (Maalox + Simethicone) 15 to 30 mL PO QID p.r.n.
   c. Psychotropic
      i. Tricyclic antidepressants (TCAs), selective serotonin reuptake inhibitors (SSRIs), anxiolytic agents (limited data for these)
3. If these attempts are unsuccessful, consider esophagogastroduodenoscopy (EGD) and treatment of *H. pylori* (see Chapter 2.45).

IV. Psychiatric pearls, pointers, and parallels
   a. Dyspepsia is more common in people who have experienced a life stressor.
   b. Depression and anxiety are more common in patients with nonulcer dyspepsia than in those with ulcers or healthy controls.
      i. Patients with nonulcer dyspepsia have more somatic symptoms than those with ulcers or healthy controls.
      ii. Nonulcer dyspepsia is more common in people who have a history of child abuse.

EAR AILMENTS

I. Cerumen mpaction
   a. General—Cerumen (earwax) tightly packed in the external ear canal and blocking the eardrum
   b. Clinical—partial hearing loss, sense of fullness in the ear, itching, tinnitus (ringing in ears), pain
   c. Etiology—usually a result of an individual unintentionally pushing cerumen into his ear
   d. Eardrop treatments (irrigation)
      i. Three percent hydrogen peroxide + water → mix 50% of each solution and apply TID
      ii. Carbamide peroxide 6.5% (Debrox) 3 to 5 drops in affected ear BID
      iii. Triethanolamine polypeptide oleate condensate (Cerumenex).
      Directions for use are as follows
         1. Fill ear canal with solution while having patient's head at 45 degrees.
         2. Insert cotton plug and allow it to remain in place for 15 to 30 minutes.
         3. Flush with lukewarm water.
II. Bacterial otitis externa (with intact tympanic membrane [TM])
   a. General—inflammation of the external ear canal with scant white mucus
   b. Clinical—otalgia (pain range: pruritis to harsh), otorrhea (discharge in/from the external ear canal)
      i. Make sure to visualize the TM to rule out otitis media.

REMEMBER:

Only attempt to clean the external ear canal of otorrhea if the TM is fully intact. Flushing the ear when the TM is not intact can cause cochlear-vestibular damage (↓ hearing, tinnitus, vertigo).

---

   c. Etiology—most common cause is bacterial (*Staphylococcus aureus, Pseudomonas*), but 10% of cases are fungal.
   d. Risk factors—moisture, mechanical removal of cerumen, insertion of foreign objects into ear, and so on.
   e. Treatment—(recommended that drops be given 3 days after symptoms end; therefore course is 7 days)
      i. Ofloxacin otic (Floxin Otic) 10 drops daily.

REMEMBER:

Ofloxacin otic 10 gtt BID × 14 days is the only topical agent with U.S. Food and Drug Administration (FDA) approval for use when the TM is perforated, although oral antibiotics are usually used.

---

    ii. Ciprofloxacin/otic (Cipro HC Otic) 3 gtt BID

    iii. Gentamicin ophthalmic (Garamycin) 3 to 4 gtt TID (The ophthalmic solution is used for ears as well)

       Note: If otitis externa is persistent, or if associated with otitis media, then use oral antibiotics (see subsequent text).

  f. Complications

    i. Necrotizing or malignant otitis externa (temporal bone osteomyelitis)

      1. General—life-threatening extension of otitis externa to mastoid or temporal bone

      2. Clinical—Otorrhea with odor

      3. Etiology—*Pseudomonas*

      4. Risk factors—old age, diabetes mellitus (DM), immuno-compromised state (e.g., human immunodeficiency virus [HIV])

      5. Treatment

        a. For mild infections, PO fluoroquinolones × 2 weeks

        b. Get ENT involved; surgical debridement may be needed

    ii. Cellulitis of the external ear

      1. Treatment—Ciprofloxacin (Cipro) 500 mg PO BID × 7 days

III. Fungal otitis externa (with intact TM)

  a. Clinical—classical result of long-term treatment of bacterial otitis externa; fluffy white discharge

  b. Etiology—Aspergillus (80%–90% of fungal cases), Candida

  c. Treatment—as with bacterial otitis externa, clear the ear canal, then

    i. Treat using any of the following; apply 3 to 4 gtt BID × 7 days

      1. Clotrimazole (Lotrimin) 1% solution

      2. Tolnaftate (Tinactin) 1% solution (can be used if TM is perforated)

      3. Itraconazole (Sporanox) (if Aspergillus is resistant to clotrimazole)

IV. Noninfectious dermatologic causes of otitis externa ("Eczematous Otitis Externa")

  a. Differential Diagnosis

    i. Atopic dermatitis (chronic, pruritic reaction to allergens or stress; family history of atopy)

    ii. Contact dermatitis (response to an irritant)

    iii. Seborrheic dermatitis (greasy or powdery scale)

    iv. Acne (open and closed comedones with pustules)

    v. Lupus (associated with discoid form of systemic lupus erythematosus [SLE])

    vi. Psoriasis (red lesions with thick, silvery adherent scale)

  b. Treatment—topical steroids

    i. Dexamethasone otic drops 3 to 4 gtt TID or QID, taper as improvement occurs.

REMEMBER:

Clear, thin, watery discharge could be from a cerebrospinal fluid (CSF) leak.

V. Otitis media

  a. General—fluid in the middle ear

  b. Classification

    i. Acute suppurative otitis media

      1. Clinical—symptoms (*bulging TM* despite positive pressure, injected, cloudy)

    ii. Otitis media with effusion

      1. Clinical—NO symptoms (TM is retracted or neutral); a form of chronic otitis media

VI. Acute suppurative otitis media

  a. Etiology—*Streptococcus pneumoniae, Haemophilus influenzae, Moraxella catarrhalis* (and their antibiotic resistant counterparts)

    i. Viruses are the sole pathogen in <10% of cases.

  b. Treatment—(challenging given plethora of antibiotic resistant strains)

    i. If NO antibiotics in the prior month

      1. Amoxicillin 500 mg PO q12h OR 875 mg PO q12h × 10 days

      2. If treatment failure on day 3, then use either:

        a. Amoxicillin/clavulanate (Augmentin) 875 mg PO q12h × 10 days

        OR Cefuroxime (Ceftin) 500 mg PO BID × 10 days

        OR Ceftriaxone (Rocephin) 1 to 2 g IM/IV daily

    ii. If antibiotic use in the prior month

      1. Use any of the following

        a. Amoxicillin 875 mg PO q12h × 10 days

        OR Amoxicillin/clavulanate 875 mg PO q12h × 10 days

        OR Cefuroxime 500 mg PO BID × 10 days

      2. If treatment failure on day 3, then use either

        a. Ceftriaxone 1 to 2 g IM/IV daily

        OR may need to perform tympanocentesis

EPILEPSY

I. Evaluation
   a. General—recurrent seizures secondary to acquired or genetic brain disorder
   b. Epidemiology—2 million in the United States have epilepsy.
   c. Diagnostic algorithm
      i. Determine whether or not the patient has seizures.
         1. Exclude migraine, syncope, transient ischemic attack, psychogenic, movement disorders, and so on.
      ii. Determine the underlying cause for seizures.
         1. Consider family history, central nervous system (CNS) trauma, sinus infection, drug abuse, cancer, and so on
         2. Complete evaluation includes electrolytes, liver function tests (LFTs), drug screen, electroencephalogram (EEG), magnetic resonance imaging (MRI), lumbar puncture. (see Table 2.26.1)

> **NOTE:**
>
> In approximately 50% of those with epilepsy, a single EEG shows no abnormalities.

II. Treatment
   a. General Guidelines
      i. Initial adverse effects include sedation, dizziness, ataxia, headache, and nausea.
         1. Adjust the dose of antiepileptics to limit toxicity and to obtain the best control of seizures.
      ii. Most antiepileptics can cause a rash which in some becomes Stevens-Johnson syndrome.
         1. Least likely to cause rash are divalproex, gabapentin, and levetiracetam
      iii. Add a second-line agent if seizures are not fully controlled with the maximum dose of the first-line agent.
      iv. If after 2 years the patient is seizure-free, withdrawal of the medication can be considered.
         1. Risk of recurrence is >50% for those with risk factors (EEG findings, etc.)
      v. In most states, licensed drivers must report a seizure condition to the Department of Motor Vehicles (DMV).
         1. Requirements are available from the Epilepsy Foundation at www.efa.org.

TABLE **2.26.1**	Evaluating Seizures		
Type of Seizure	**Clinical Features**	**EEG Findings**	**Treatment**
Simple partial seizure	Focal electrical discharge causing motor, sensory, autonomic, or psychic symptoms; patient remains conscious	Focal slowing, sharp-wave activity, or both	Oxcarbazepine (Trileptal) Carbamazepine (Tegretol) Phenytoin (Dilantin) Divalproex (Depakote)
Complex partial seizure (temporal lobe seizures, psychomotor seizures)	May be preceded by a simple partial seizure; consciousness impaired; automatisms (repetitive behaviors of which the patient has no recollection); post-ictal confusion	Focal slowing, sharp-wave activity, or both	Oxcarbazepine (Trileptal) Carbamazepine (Tegretol) Phenytoin (Dilantin) Divalproex (Depakote)
Absence seizure (petit mal)	Seizure begins rapidly with approximately 10 sec of unresponsiveness and rapid recovery; may or may not have changes in muscle tone, automatisms, or clonic movement.	Spike-wave pattern (3 Hz)	Ethosuximide (Zarontin) Divalproex (Depakote)
Generalized tonic–clonic seizure (grand mal)	Loss of consciousness; tonic increase in muscle tone followed by clonic jerks; patient is comatose after seizure and improves slowly; incontinence and tongue biting may occur.	Spike-wave pattern (3–5 Hz)	Divalproex (Depakote) Phenytoin (Dilantin)

Simple = consciousness not impaired; Complex = consciousness impaired; Partial = only part of the cortex is involved at the seizure's onset.
EEG, electroencephalogram.
Adapted from Browne TR, Holmes GL. Epilepsy. *N Engl J Med.* 2001;344(15):1145–1151.

   b. First-line medications
      i. Oxcarbazepine (Trileptal) 300 mg PO BID
         1. Maintenance = 600 to 2,400 mg per day; maximum = 2,400 mg per day
         2. Therapeutic range—not established

  ii. Carbamazepine (Tegretol) 200 mg PO BID
   1. Maintenance = 600 to 1,200 mg per day; maximum = 1,600 mg per day, keeping within therapeutic range
   2. Therapeutic range—4 to 12 μg per mL
  iii. Phenytoin (Dilantin) 300 mg PO daily
   1. Maintenance = 300 to 500 mg per day
   2. Therapeutic range = 10 to 20 μg per mL
    a. At levels >10, a change in dose has a disproportionate effect
     i. Therefore, only increase or decrease the dose by 30 to 50 mg when level is >10.
   3. Special considerations
    a. Loading dose = 400 mg PO, followed by 300 mg × 2, at 2-hour intervals
    b. Phenytoin toxicity (death can result from respiratory or cardiovascular collapse)
     i. Dizziness, confusion, ataxia, tremor, nystagmus, blurry vision
     ii. Dysarthria or slurred speech
     iii. Nausea, vomiting
     iv. Hyperreflexia
     v. Hypotension
  iv. Divalproex (Depakote) 250 to 500 mg PO BID.
   1. Maintenance = 1 to 3 g per day; Maximum 60 mg/kg/day, keeping within therapeutic range
   2. Therapeutic range: 50 to 150 μg per mL
  v. Ethosuximide (Zarontin) 250 mg PO BID
   1. Maintenance = 1,000 to 2,000 mg per day
   2. Therapeutic range: 40 to 120 μg per mL
 c. Adjunctive medications (see Table 2.26.2)
III. Status epilepticus
 a. General—two or more sequential seizures without full recovery of consciousness between seizures
  OR >30 minutes of unremitting seizure activity
 b. Etiology—noncompliance, alcohol withdrawal, CNS infection, metabolic causes, and so on
 c. Management—activate Emergency Medical Services (EMS) as this is a medical emergency
  i. ABCs (*A*irway, *B*reathing, *C*irculation)—oxygen, intubate if needed to protect airway, neuro examination
  ii. Laboratories—electrolytes, blood urea nitrogen (BUN), glucose, complete blood count (CBC), drug screen, anticonvulsant levels, arterial blood gas (ABG)
  iii. Start an IV; give 50 mL of 50% glucose IV and 100 mg of thiamine IV/IM
  iv. Obtain an EEG
  v. Medications (continue down the list if seizures persist)

TABLE **2.26.2**	Adjunctive Medications		
Medication	**Starting Dose**	**Maintenance Dose**	**Therapeutic Range**
Gabapentin (Neurontin)	300 mg PO TID.	900–3,600 mg/d	Not established
Lamotrigine (Lamictal)	25 mg PO daily	300–500 mg/d	Not established
Levetiracetam (Keppra)	500 mg PO BID.	1,000–3,000 mg/d	Not established
Phenobarbital	90 mg PO daily	90–120 mg/d	10–40 μg/mL
Primidone (Mysoline)	100 mg PO qhs–TID.	750–1,000 mg/d	5–12 μg/mL
Tiagabine (Gabitril)	2 mg PO BID.	32–56 mg/d	Not established
Topiramate (Topamax)	25 mg PO qhs–BID.	200–400 mg/d	Not established
Zonisamide (Zonegran)	50 mg PO BID.	400–600 mg/d	Not established

Adapted from Browne TR, Holmes GL. Epilepsy. *N Engl J Med.* 2001;344(15):1145–1151, with additional information from Micromedex, http://www.micromedex.com.

1. Lorazepam (Ativan) 0.1 to 0.15 mg per kg IV (2 mg/minute)
2. Fosphenytoin (Cerebyx) 18 to 25 mg per kg IV (150 mg/minute)
3. Phenobarbital 20 mg per kg IV (100 mg/minute) loading dose
4. Pentobarbital IV drip
   OR Midazolam (Versed) IV drip
   OR Propofol (Diprivan) IV drip

IV. Psychiatric pearls, pointers, and parallels
   a. Nonepileptic seizures (NES)

REMEMBER:

Many patients with NES also have epileptic seizures, and therefore, they may require antiepileptic medications.

---

     i. Clinical—symptoms of NES are similar to epileptic seizures.
    ii. Etiology—nonepileptic seizures are not caused by electrical disruptions in the brain, as with epilepsy.
      1. Subtypes
        a. Physiologic NES
          i. Owing to physical or chemical factors
            1. For example, infection, hypoglycemia, alcohol withdrawal, arrhythmia, and so on
        b. Psychogenic NES

i. Owing to stressful events, including psychological distress or trauma
- iii. Epidemiology
    1. Up to 20% of patients with epilepsy actually have NES.
    2. Ten percent of patients with NES also have epileptic seizures.
- iv. Diagnosis
    1. Rule out epileptic seizures.
    2. Video EEG is the gold standard for diagnosis.
- v. Treatment
    1. Antiepileptic medications are not helpful.
    2. Treat depression and anxiety, as they are often the primary problems for these patients.

2.27

EPISTAXIS (NOSEBLEED)

I. Evaluation
- a. General—nosebleeds occur in up to 60% of people over a lifetime; 6% require medical care.
- b. Etiology—(environmental factors, i.e., humidity, temperature, and altitude also require consideration.)
    - i. Local causes
        1. Idiopathic (80%–90%)
        2. Trauma—epistaxis digitorum (nose picking), facial injury, foreign body
        3. Inflammation—infection (e.g., sinusitis), allergies
        4. Neoplasia and/or nasal polyps
        5. Vascular malformation
        6. Structural—septal deviation or perforation
        7. Drugs—medications (e.g., nasal sprays—decongestants, corticosteroids), cocaine
    - ii. Systemic causes
        1. Hematologic—coagulopathies, low platelet count, or platelet dysfunction
        2. Medications—anticoagulants (e.g., warfarin), antiplatelet agents (e.g., aspirin)
        3. Liver disease (e.g., cirrhosis)
        4. Hypertension
- c. Epidemiology—bimodal distribution (peaks at younger than 10 years of age and older than 50 years); ♂ > ♀

d. Classification
   i. Anatomy
      1. Anterior epistaxis (80% of epistaxis)
         a. Clinical—nasal bleeding is obvious.
         b. Mechanism—bleeding arises from Kiesselbach's plexus.
      2. Posterior epistaxis
         a. Clinical—may be asymptomatic or can present insidiously.
         b. Mechanism—bleeding arises from branches of the sphenopalatine artery.

REMEMBER:

Epistaxis is potentially life threatening.

II. Management
   a. Initial treatment
      i. Nasal maneuvers
         1. Apply direct pressure to the septum to compress the nostrils (5–20 minutes).
         2. Plug the affected nostril with gauze/cotton.
         3. Tilt head forward; this precludes blood from collecting in the posterior pharynx.
      ii. Fluid management
         1. Monitor vital signs regularly.
         2. If volume depletion is present, then give fluids; type and screen the patient's blood.
   b. Additional treatment when bleeding continues despite compression and nasal plugging
      i. Consider a systemic process if bleeding is diffuse, occurs at multiple sites, or is recurrent.
         1. Hematologic evaluation—complete blood counts (CBC), prothrombin time (PT)/international normalized ratio (INR), partial thromboplastin time (PTT)
      ii. Locate the source of bleeding.
         1. Anterior epistaxis
            a. Increase visibility by having the patient take a forceful blow to clear clots; apply a local anesthetic and attempt vasoconstriction for a single site.
               i. Lidocaine injection 0.5% to 2% + epinephrine 1/200,000
               ii. Lidocaine topical 5% + phenylephrine nasal 0.125% to 0.5%
            b. If unsuccessful, chemical cautery can be tried using silver nitrate.
               i. Apply silver nitrate to bleeding site for 30 seconds.
               ii. Can also consider electrocautery (performed by otolaryngologist).

      c. If unsuccessful, then perform nasal packing with ribbon gauze or nasal tampons.
- i. Apply topical antibiotic (Neosporin) to packing materials.
- ii. Nasal packing may remain in place for 3 to 5 days.

    2. Posterior epistaxis
- a. Difficult to treat; typically treated by otolaryngologist.
- b. Usually requires balloon insertion or a posterior pack.

  c. Further treatment for persistent bleeding despite the aforementioned interventions
- i. May necessitate hot water irrigation, surgery, arterial ligation, or embolization

  d. Future precautions after episode of epistaxis resolves
- i. Avoid spicy foods and cigarettes to prevent vasodilation.
- ii. Avoid vigorous exercise for a few days.
- iii. Modify environmental factors (if possible)—that is, humidity, temperature, and altitude.

2.28

FOOT AILMENTS

I. Callus (calluses)
- a. General—thickening of the outermost layer of the skin as a result of repeated pressure/friction
- b. Clinical—pain results as the callus thickens and causes more pressure against the underlying skin
- c. Treatment
  - i. Soak feet in warm water (with one to two capfuls of bleach) for 15 minutes; rub off dead skin
    OR Dr. Scholl's salicylic acid containing products; apply as directed.
  - ii. Prevention! (Avoid poor-fitting shoes.)

II. Clavus (clavi) ("corns")
- a. General—develops like a callus, but its central aspect is hyperkeratotic and painful.
- b. Clinical—typically occurs at pressure points (i.e., a result of poor-fitting shoes).
- c. Treatment—same as with callus.

III. Painful feet
- a. General—may result from long walks, blisters, cracks, and so on

b. Treatment
   i. Soak feet in warm water with povidone-iodine (Betadine) for 15 minutes BID.
   ii. If cracks are deep, place an antibiotic ointment after foot is soaked BID.

IV. Plantar warts
   a. General—a benign neoplasm of the skin caused by human papillomavirus (HPV)
   b. Clinical—often occur at pressure points; may cause pain when walking
      i. Sometimes mistaken for clavi
   c. Treatment
      i. Soak wart in warm water for 5 minutes, remove tissue if possible, and dry.
      ii. Then apply salicyclic acid to the affected area BID for a maximum of 12 weeks.

V. Tinea unguium (onychomycosis)
   a. General—fungal infection of the toenails/fingernails
   b. Clinical—nail is thick, brittle, hard, and discolored (yellow/brown); often associated with tinea pedis (see Chapter 2.54)
   c. Etiology—*Trichophyton rubrum*, a dermatophyte, accounts for 80% of all nail fungal infections; *Trichophyton mentagrophytes*
   d. Epidemiology—approximately 2% of the US population
   e. Treatment
      i. Topical
         1. Miconazole topical 2% powder applied BID over nail plate
         2. Clotrimazole topical 1% cream applied BID.
         3. Ciclopirox (Penlac Nail Lacquer) 8%—apply to nail qhs (maximum 48 weeks).
      ii. Oral (use these medications with caution—monitor liver function tests (LFTs), avoid with pregnancy, etc.)
         1. Itraconazole (Sporanox) 200 mg PO daily × 3 months
         2. Terbinafine (Lamisil) 250 mg PO daily × 6 weeks (fingernails)
            Terbinafine (Lamisil) 250 mg PO daily × 12 weeks (toenails)
         3. Fluconazole (Diflucan) 150 to 300 mg every week until infection clears

VI. Tinea pedis ("athlete's foot") (see Chapter 2.54)
   a. General—dermatophyte infection of the feet; most common dermatophyte infection
   b. Clinical—erythematous scaling plaques, pruritis, presents as a
      i. Maceration between the toes (toe-web distribution)
         OR diffuse erythema affecting the soles (moccasin distribution)
   c. Etiology—most commonly caused by the dermatophytes *T. rubrum* and mentagrophytes

    d. Risk factors—occlusive footwear
    e. Treatment
      i. Topical—apply medication to include skin approximately 2 cm beyond the affected area.
        1. Butenafine (Mentax, Lotrimin Ultra)—apply daily × 4 weeks
          OR Butenafine (Mentax, Lotrimin Ultra)—apply BID. × 1 week
        2. Azole—clotrimazole (Lotrimin AF, Mycelex) topical 1% cream—apply BID for up to 4 weeks.
        3. Tolnaftate (Tinactin) topical 1% cream—apply BID up to 4 to 6 weeks.
        4. Naftifine (Naftin) 1% cream daily for up to 4 weeks.
      ii. Combination topical treatment
        1. Betamethasone/clotrimazole (Lotrisone) topical 0.05%/1% cream—apply BID up to 4 weeks.
      iii. Systemic treatment
        1. Allylamine—terbinafine (Lamisil) 250 mg PO daily × 2 weeks
        2. Triazole—itraconazole (Sporanox) 200 mg PO BID × 2 weeks
          a. Adverse effect—reversible hepatitis, so watch LFTs.
    f. Prevention
      i. Use foot powder that absorbs moisture.
      ii. Frequently change of socks and shoes (do not allow feet to become moist).

2.29

GASTROESOPHAGEAL REFLUX DISEASE

I. Evaluation
    a. General—a common, chronic condition characterized by heartburn once or more in a month
    b. Clinical:
      i. Classic symptoms → acid regurgitation and heartburn
      ii. Atypical symptoms → asthma, chest pain, cough, dental caries, laryngitis, and sore throat

   c. Epidemiology—44% of US adults have heartburn

   d. Risk factors (of complicated gastroesophageal reflux disease [GERD]):

      i. Dysphagia, odynophagia (painful swallowing), bleeding, emesis, decrease in weight, early satiety

      ii. Risk factors for Barrett's esophagus—white, male, aged 45 or older, long-standing symptom duration

   e. Diagnosis

      i. Empiric acid suppression × 4 to 8 weeks for those with typical symptoms and no risk factors

         1. If this resolves the patient's ailment, then there is no need for a 24-hour pH probe.

      ii. For those with possible esophageal complications/Barrett's, get an esophagogastroduodenoscopy (EGD)

II. Treatment

   a. Lifestyle modifications

      i. Avoid large meals, acidic foods, alcohol, and caffeine.

      ii. Avoid wearing clothing that is too tight around the waist.

      iii. Avoid lying down within 4 hours of a meal.

      iv. Decrease dietary fat intake and lose weight.

      v. Raise the head of the bed.

      vi. Smoking cessation.

   b. Medications (can employ "step-up" or "step-down" therapy; usually treat for 8 weeks)

REMEMBER:

"Step-up" therapy begins with 8 weeks of a histamine H_2-antagonist, and progresses to a proton pump inhibitor (PPI) if symptoms are not relieved; "step-down" therapy begins with 8 weeks of a PPI, and downgrades medication and dosage to lowest effective dose.

---

      i. Antacids—occasional heartburn responds well to antacids

         1. Maalox (aluminum and magnesium hydroxide) 15 to 30 mL PO QID p.r.n.

         2. Mylanta (Maalox + Simethicone) 15 to 30 mL PO QID p.r.n.

         3. Sucralfate (Carafate) 1 g PO QID (1 hour before meals and qhs)

      ii. H_2-receptor antagonists—up to 70% of patients report relief

         1. Cimetidine (Tagamet) 400 to 800 mg PO BID

            a. Lots of drug–drug interactions because it is a cytochrome P450 inhibitor

         2. Famotidine (Pepcid) 20 to 40 mg PO/IV BID

         3. Ranitidine (Zantac) 150 mg PO BID

         4. Nizatidine (Axid) 150 mg PO BID

       iii. PPI—provides most control of reflux symptoms
1. Rabeprazole (Aciphex) 20 mg PO daily to BID
2. Lansoprazole (Prevacid) 15 to 30 mg PO daily to BID
3. Pantoprazole (Protonix) 40 mg PO/IV daily to BID
4. Omeprazole (Prilosec) 20 to 80 mg PO daily
5. Esomeprazole (Nexium) 20 to 40 mg PO/IV daily to BID
  c. Antireflux surgery
    i. Even within 3 to 5 years of surgery, approximately 50% are taking antireflux medications again.

2.30

GLAUCOMA, OPEN-ANGLE

I. Evaluation
  a. General—an optic neuropathy that leads to death of optic nerve tissue; decrease in peripheral vision
  b. Clinical—progressive disease of the optic nerve with an increase in intraocular pressure (IOP) and optic disc cupping
    i. Peripheral vision gradually declines, is asymptomatic, and is irreversible.

> **REMEMBER:**
>
> A painful red eye associated with nausea/vomiting implies acute angle-closure glaucoma until proved otherwise.

  c. Mechanism—impaired outflow of aqueous humor results in increased IOP (>21 mm Hg); gradually, optic nerve cells die leading to enlargement of the optic nerve cup (cup-to-disc >0.5)

> **REMEMBER:**
>
> In angle-closure glaucoma, the anterior chamber angle becomes occluded resulting in blockage of aqueous outflow; IOP rises quickly and vision loss from ischemia can occur within hours. Hence, a medical emergency.

  d. Epidemiology—3% of those aged older than 55 years in the United States have glaucoma; $>90\%$ of cases are open angle
  e. Risk factors—old age, African American, family history, increased IOP, topical eye steroids
  f. Diagnostic algorithm—those with risk factors or clinical findings should go to ophthalmology

      i.   Perimetry displays a printout of visual fields.

II. Treatment

  a. Nonpharmacologic management

      i.   Aerobic exercise can lower IOP.

  b. Pharmacologic management

      i. β-Blockers, nonspecific—decrease aqueous production (formerly the first drug class chosen)

        1. Timolol ophthalmic (Timoptic) 0.5%—1 gtt OS/OD daily to BID

        2. Levobunolol ophthalmic (Betagan) 0.5%—1 gtt OS/OD daily to BID

        Side effects: Cardiac ($\downarrow$ heart rate [HR], $\downarrow$ blood pressure [BP], heart block, worsened congestive heart failure [CHF]), bronchospasm

     ii. β-Blockers, relatively specific—decrease aqueous production

        1. Betaxolol ophthalmic (Betoptic S) 0.25%—1 to 2 gtt OS/OD BID

        Side effects: Less risk of systemic side effects, especially pulmonary

   iii. Carbonic anhydrase inhibitors—decrease aqueous production (often adjunctive therapy)

        1. Dorzolamide ophthalmic (Trusopt) 2%—1 gtt OS/OD TID

        2. Brinzolamide ophthalmic (Azopt) 1%—1 gtt OS/OD TID

        Side effects: Malaise, weight loss, depressed mood, gastrointestinal (GI) cramps, nephrolithiasis, and dyscrasias

   iv. α_2-Agonists—decrease aqueous production, increase outflow (primary or adjunctive therapy)

        1. Apraclonidine ophthalmic (Iopidine) 0.5%—1 gtt OS/OD BID to TID

        2. Brimonidine ophthalmic (Alphagan P) 0.1%—1 gtt OS/OD TID

        Side effects: No cardiovascular side effects with apraclonidine, but hypotension with brimonidine

    v. Sympathomimetic—increase aqueous outflow (rarely used)

        1. Dipivefrin ophthalmic (Propine) 0.1%—1 gtt OS/OD q12h

        Side effects: Limited systemic side effects, but many ocular side effects

   vi. Prostaglandin analogs—increase aqueous outflow (most frequently prescribed in the world)

        1. Latanoprost ophthalmic (Xalatan) 0.005%—1 gtt OS/OD every evening

        2. Travoprost ophthalmic (Travatan) 0.004%—1 gtt OS/OD every evening

        Side effects: Iris darkens in 10% of patients, eyelashes become longer

vii. Parasympathomimetic—increase aqueous outflow
  1. Pilocarpine ophthalmic (Pilocar) 1% to 4% solution 1 to 2 gtt OS/OD TID to QID
     Side effects: Fixed, small pupils; myopia
viii. Combination medication
  1. Dorzolamide/Timolol (Cosopt) 2/0.5%—1 gtt OS/OD BID
c. Surgical management (laser trabeculoplasty OR surgical trabeculectomy)
  i. For those who have progressive optic nerve damage and cannot achieve the goal IOP medically

2.31

GOUT

I. Evaluation
  a. General—inflammatory response to monosodium urate crystal deposition in joint(s)
  b. Clinical
     i. Acute—often begins at night with intense pain, redness, swelling, warmth, and decreased movement.
       1. Affects first metatarsophalangeal joint in >70% of cases; also tarsal joints, ankles, knees, wrists.
       2. Usually monoarticular, but can be polyarticular (if so, fever is more likely).
     ii. Chronic—after approximately 10 years, the tophaceous phase occurs.
  c. Mechanism
     i. Hyperuricemia—secondary to
       1. Insufficient renal excretion
         a. Genetic predisposition (e.g., rare enzyme defects)
         b. Chronic renal failure
         c. Medications—loop or thiazide diuretics, low dose aspirin, cyclosporine
       2. Urate overproduction
         a. Urate rich food (meats—beef, pork, lamb)
         b. Excess alcohol
         c. Obesity (with insulin resistance) and decreased physical activity
         d. Diseases of increased cell turnover (e.g., myeloproliferative or lymphoproliferative)

NOTE:

Hyperuricemia is often associated with the metabolic syndrome (hypertension [HTN], diabetes mellitus [DM], ↑ triglycerides [TG], obesity).

d. Epidemiology—♂:♀ is approximately 8:1; men after age 35, women after age 65
e. Diagnostic algorithm
   i. Diagnostic—joint aspiration showing needle shaped, negatively birefringent urate crystals
   ii. Suggestive—increased serum urate concentration (≥9 mg/dL)

REMEMBER:

Do not forget to rule out *septic arthritis*—letting this disease go untreated can be devastating. Also, rule out *pseudogout* (elderly, affects knees or wrists, chondrocalcinosis, pyrophosphate crystals in joint).

II. Treatment
   a. Nonsteroidal anti-inflammatory drugs (NSAIDS)—no difference in efficacy amongst NSAIDS; treat for 5 to 7 days.
      i. Naproxen (Naprosyn) 250 to 500 mg PO BID
      ii. Indomethacin (Indocin) 50 mg PO TID
      iii. Celecoxib (Celebrex) 400 mg PO on day 1, then 200 mg PO daily

REMEMBER:

Avoid aspirin because at low doses it can cause the kidneys to retain uric acid.

   b. Colchicine—inhibits urate crystal phagocytosis, so it is most effective early after symptom onset.
      i. Colchicine 0.6 mg PO q1h for up to 3 hours
      ii. Prophylactic dosing—Colchicine 0.6 mg PO every other day–BID
      iii. Adverse effects—diarrhea, emesis (occur quickly given narrow therapeutic index)
      iv. Note—be careful with poor renal clearance and with the elderly
   c. Intra-articular corticosteroids—for medium or large sized joints in absence of septic arthritis.
      i. Methylprednisolone 40 mg (for medium joints), 80 mg (for large joints)
   d. System corticosteroids—for multiple joints or when intra-articular therapy is not feasible.
      i. Prednisone 40 to 60 mg PO × 3 days, then decrease by 10 mg per day q3d until complete

III. Prophylaxis

> **NOTE:**
>
> Sixty-two percent of patients have a recurrent gouty flair within 1 year.

    a. Correctable risk factors—decrease meat consumption, decrease alcohol, find an alternative to diuretic therapy

    b. Allopurinol (Zyloprim) 50 to 300 mg PO daily

       i. Titration—start low (100 mg daily) and increase every few weeks until serum urate normalizes.

          1. Note—be careful with dosage, as it is based on creatinine clearance

       ii. Adverse effects—severe hypersensitivity syndrome, mild rash, precipitation of acute gout

    c. Probenecid 250 mg PO BID, and gradually increase to 500 to 1,000 mg PO BID until urate is <6

       i. Adverse effects—urolithiasis, impairment of renal function, precipitation of acute gout

    d. Sulfinpyrazone (Anturane) 50 mg PO BID, and gradually increase to 100 to 400 mg PO BID until urate is <6.

       i. Adverse effects—urolithiasis, impairment of renal function, precipitation of acute gout

IV. Psychiatric pearls, pointers, and parallels

    a. Allopurinol

       i. Some clinical trials have shown that allopurinol may have antiaggression properties.

          1. There may be a role (although data is limited) for purines in the development of schizophrenia.

             a. Some data shows allopurinol can be an adjuvant treatment for refractory schizophrenia.

          2. There are case reports of allopurinol use in acute manic episodes.

          3. There are also case reports of allopurinol use in the treatment of aggression in patients with dementia.

       ii. Further controlled studies are needed due to lack of evidence-based data for these uses of allopurinol.

    b. NSAIDS

       i. There are a few case reports of NSAID-induced psychosis, which resolved on withdrawal of the NSAID

HEADACHES (CEPHALALGIA)

I. Evaluation
   a. General—pain affecting the head, although typically not confined to a particular nerve distribution
   b. Classification
      i. Common primary headache disorders
         1. Tension-type headache
         2. Migraine headache
         3. Cluster headache
      ii. Secondary headache disorders
         1. Vascular (e.g., subarachnoid hemorrhage, stroke, arteritis, arteriovenous [AV] malformation, etc.)
         2. Intracranial (e.g., neoplasm, pseudotumor cerebri, infection, posttrauma, etc.)
         3. Metabolic (e.g., hypoglycemia, hypoxia, hypercapnia, dialysis, etc.)
         4. Myofascial (e.g., cervical spine disorders, etc.)
         5. Sleep disorders (e.g., obstructive sleep apnea)
         6. Substance use or withdrawal
   c. Diagnostic algorithm
      i. Initial task—rule out a potentially life-threatening etiology for the patient's headache.
         1. Signs/symptoms of concern (see Table 2.32.1)
II. Common primary headaches and acute management
   a. Tension-type headache
      i. Clinical—bilateral, band-like pressure around the head with varying location and intensity
         1. Attacks last 30 minutes to 7 days (sometimes months in extreme cases).
         2. It is associated with tightness of the neck and shoulders.
         3. There is no nausea, vomiting, aura, or photophobia.
      ii. Etiology—usually results from stress (emotional upset)
         1. Associated with physical causes (muscle strain/tension of the neck and shoulders)
      iii. Treatment
         1. Nonpharmacologic
            a. Stress avoidance, stretching, relaxation exercises, physical therapy, and so on
         2. Pharmacologic options for abortive therapy (i.e., acute treatment)

TABLE **2.32.1**	Headache Signs and Symptoms	
Symptom of Clinical Concern	**Differential Diagnosis**	**Possible Evaluation**
Late onset (first headache after age 50)	Mass lesion Temporal arteritis	Neuroimaging ESR, biopsy
"Worst headache of my life!"	Subarachnoid hemorrhage	Neuroimaging; may need LP if neuroimaging is negative and clinical suspicion is high
Sudden onset of headache	Mass lesion or hemorrhage into mass lesion Subarachnoid hemorrhage AV malformation Pituitary apoplexy (hemorrhage/infarction of pituitary)	Neuroimaging; may need LP if neuroimaging is negative and clinical suspicion is high
Worsening headache (changes in character of headache)	Mass lesion Subdural hematoma Medication overuse	Neuroimaging Drug screen
Headache following trauma	Hemorrhage (intracranial, epidural, or subdural) Posttraumatic headache	Neuroimaging May need to image cervical spine
Headache associated with signs of infection	Infectious etiology (local or systemic)	Neuroimaging; LP with serology
New headache in patient with HIV	Local infection vs. abscess	Neuroimaging; LP vs. brain biopsy
New headache in cancer patient	Metastasis	Neuroimaging; may need LP if neuroimaging is negative and clinical suspicion is high
Focal neurologic signs	Mass lesion (may have papilledema) Pseudotumor cerebri (papilledema) Stroke or AV malformation	Neuroimaging; may need LP

ESR, erythrocyte sedimentation rate; LP, lumbar puncture; AV, arteriovenous; HIV, human immunodeficiency virus.
Adapted from Newman LC, Lipton RB. Emergency department evaluation of headache. *Neurol Clin.* 1998;16:285–303, with additional information from Clinch CR. Evaluation of acute headaches in adults. *Am Fam Physician.* 2001;63(4):685–692.

> **REMEMBER:**
>
> Medications work best acutely when given as soon as the headache (tension, migraine, or cluster) is recognized.

    a. Nonsteroidal anti-inflammatory drugs (NSAIDS) (avoid in those with gastrointestinal [GI] or bleeding disorders)

       i. Naproxen (Naprosyn) 250 to 500 mg PO BID

    b. Muscle relaxants

       i. Cyclobenzaprine (Flexeril) 5 to 10 mg PO TID.

       ii. Diazepam (Valium) 2 to 10 mg PO BID to QID

    c. Combination analgesics

       i. Midrin 325/100/65—take one to two capsules PO q6h. Midrin is composed of:

         1. Acetaminophen 325 mg

         2. Dichloralphenazone 100 mg—an anxiolytic

         3. Isometheptene 65 mg—a sympathomimetic

       ii. Fioricet 325/50/40—take one to two tablets PO q8h. Fioricet is composed of:

         1. Acetaminophen 325 mg

         2. Butalbital 50 mg—a barbiturate (abusable agent)

         3. Caffeine 40 mg—a stimulant

b. Migraine headache

    i. Clinical—unilateral (or sometimes bilateral) pulsating headache lasting 4 to 72 hours

       1. It is associated with nausea, vomiting, photophobia, and/or phonophobia.

       2. Can be worsened by physical activity as mild as walking stairs.

       3. Patients try to lie still in a dark room in order to get comfortable.

    ii. Mechanism—disturbance in serotonin activity in the central nervous system (CNS) with cerebral vascular dilation

    iii. Etiology—genetic

    iv. Epidemiology—3♀ : 1♂ in adults; affects 10% of Americans

    v. Precipitants—foods (e.g., chocolate), alcohol, stress, odors, exertion, hormonal changes, and so on

    vi. Classification

       1. Migraine with aura (formerly classic migraine)

         a. General—an aura is a short-lived (10–30 minutes) neurologic process.

           i. Auras are usually visual (tunnel vision, scotoma, etc.)

       2. Migraine without aura (formerly common migraine)

         a. General—occur gradually or present on waking from sleep

vii. Treatment
   1. Nonpharmacologic
      a. Stress reduction, stretching, limit/eliminate precipitating factors, and so on
   2. Pharmacologic options for abortive therapy (i.e., acute treatment)

NOTE:

Antiemetics can improve absorption of analgesic medications and therefore the two are sometimes given in combination.

---

      a. NSAIDS (avoid in those with GI or bleeding disorders)
         i. Naproxen (Naprosyn) 250 to 500 mg PO BID
            Aspirin 900 mg PO q6h
      b. Acetaminophen (Tylenol) 1,000 mg PO q6h
      c. Ergotamines—act as vasoconstrictors; can cause peripheral ischemia
         i. Cafergot (Ergotamine/caffeine)—take 1 to 2 PO q30min × 2
            Cafergot suppository—take 1 PR q30min × 2 (maximum)
         ii. Dihydroergotamine (DHE 45) 1 mg IM/IV, up to 3 mg/attack
            Nasal preparation = Migranal one spray each nostril q15min × 2
            NOTE: Do NOT use ergotamines more than every 5 days, as frequent ergotamine use leads to rebound headaches
      d. Isometheptene
         i. Midrin—take one to two capsules PO q1h, up to five capsules q12h
      e. Triptans act as vasoconstrictors; avoid in those with ischemic disease (see Table 2.32.2)

Contraindicated in those with ischemic heart disease, cerebrovascular disease, and uncontrolled hypertension. Avoid with patients taking monoamine oxidase inhibitors (MAOIs), selective serotonin reuptake inhibitors (SSRIs), and St. John's wort as serotonin syndrome may occur

   c. Cluster headache
      i. Clinical—severe, rapid unilateral pain affecting orbital/temporal areas; lasts 15 to 180 minutes
         1. It is associated with scleral injection, lacrimation, congestion, rhinorrhea, ptosis, and so on.
         2. Patients try to move about in an attempt to get comfortable (as in colic).
         3. Cyclic attacks occurring daily for weeks to months and then disappearing for months to years.

TABLE 2.32.2 Triptans

Medication (Maximum dose in a 24-hr period)	Half-life (hr)
Sumatriptan (Imitrex) 25–100 mg PO q2h × 2 [200 mg]	2
Sumatriptan nasal (Imitrex nasal) 5 or 20 mg in one nostril q2h × 2 [40 mg]	
Sumatriptan injection (Imitrex) 6 mg SC q1h × 2 [12 mg]	
Rizatriptan (Maxalt) 5–10 mg PO/ODT q2h × 3 [30 mg]	2
Zolmitriptan (Zomig) 1.25–2.5 mg PO/ODT q2h × 2 [10 mg]	3
Zolmitriptan nasal (Zomig nasal) 5 mg in one nostril q2h × 2 [10 mg]	
Almotriptan (Axert) 6.25–12.5 mg PO q2h × 2 [25 mg]	3.5
Eletriptan (Relpax) 20–40 mg PO q2h × 2 [80 mg]	5
Naratriptan (Amerge) 1–2.5 mg PO q4h × 2 [5 mg]	5—6.3
Frovatriptan (Frova) 2.5 mg PO q2h × 2 [7.5 mg]	25

ODT, orally disintegrating tablets.
Adapted from Goadsby PJ, Lipton RB, Ferrari MD. Migraine—current understanding and treatment. *N Eng J Med.* 2002;346(4):257–70, with additional information from Micromedex, http://www.micromedex.com.

      ii. Etiology—smoking, alcohol, and stress all contribute to cluster headaches
         1. Some report head trauma even months before the onset of cluster headaches.
      iii. Epidemiology—6 ♂ : 1♀; affects <0.5% of Americans
         1. Typically has an onset later in life (>30 years old)
      iv. Treatment
         1. Nonpharmacologic
            a. Stress reduction, smoking cessation, abstinence from alcohol
         2. Pharmacologic options for abortive therapy (i.e., acute treatment)
            a. Limited options; onset of headache is rapid and relatively short-lived.
            b. Oxygen 6L through facial mask terminates cluster headaches in most patients.
            c. Some patients have success with DHE 45 or the triptans.
III. Chronic daily headaches and preventive management
    a. General—headache for >15 days per month for a period of >3 months
    b. Epidemiology—3% to 5% of the world's population
    c. Risk factors—obesity, caffeine consumption, overuse of medications for acute headache, and so on

---

NOTE:

Greater than 50% of those with chronic daily headaches have concomitant mood disorders and sleep disturbances.

d. Classification—(most common)
   i. Medication-overuse headache
   ii. Chronic tension-type headache
   iii. Transformed migraine headache
   iv. Cluster headache
e. Preventive treatments
   i. Nonpharmacologic (Lifestyle modifications)
      1. Limit/eliminate caffeine
      2. Regular exercise
      3. Regular mealtimes and sleep schedules
      4. Relaxation techniques and biofeedback
   ii. Pharmacologic options for prophylactic/preventive therapy
       (i.e., chronic treatment)
       1. Antidepressants
          a. Tricyclic antidepressants (TCAs) such as Amitriptyline
             (Elavil) 50 to 100 mg PO qhs
          b. SSRIs such as Fluoxetine (Prozac) 20 to 60 mg PO
             daily
       2. Anticonvulsants
          a. Divalproex (Depakote) 250 to 1,000 mg PO BID
          b. Gabapentin (Neurontin) 300 to 1,200 mg PO TID
          c. Topiramate (Topamax) 50 to 100 mg PO BID
       3. β-blockers
          a. Propranolol (Inderal) 40 to 120 mg PO BID
          b. Metoprolol (Lopressor) 50 to 100 mg PO BID
       4. α_2-adrenergic agonists
          a. Tizanidine (Zanaflex) 2 to 4 mg PO TID
          b. Clonidine (Catapres) 0.1 to 0.3 mg PO BID
       5. Calcium-channel blockers
          a. Verapamil (Calan/Isoptin) 80 mg PO TID
       6. Antihistamines
          a. Cyproheptadine 4 mg PO TID
       7. Neurotoxin
          a. Botulinum toxin type A 25 to 260 units q3mo

REMEMBER:

There is low efficacy from long-term opioids in managing chronic headaches;
furthermore, abuse potential is high.

---

   iii. Additional options for cluster headache (not U.S. Food and
        Drug Administration [FDA] approved)
        1. Lithium (Eskalith) 300 to 600 mg PO BID
        2. Prednisone 100 mg PO daily with taper to discontinuation
   iv. Strategies for treating medication-overuse headaches
       1. Use preventive medications as listed in the preceding text
          and withdraw overused medications.

a. NSAIDs and ergotamines can be used for breakthrough headaches.

REMEMBER:

Withdrawal from analgesics and ergotamines can cause severe headache, GI side effects, hypotension, and tachycardia that can last days to weeks.

---

b. If withdrawal effects occur, consider Prednisone 100 mg PO daily × 5 days.

IV. Psychiatric pearls, pointers, and parallels
   a. When evaluating the patient with headaches, psychiatric etiologies include the following
      i. Affective disorders
      ii. Anxiety disorders
      iii. Somatoform disorders—headache is often a complaint
      iv. Drug-induced—alcohol, caffeine, drugs of abuse, medications, and so on
      v. Drug-withdrawal—rebound phenomena
   b. Management of headaches in affective disorders
      i. Depression and headaches—consider treatment with an SSRI, serotonin norepinephrine reuptake inhibitor (SNRI), or TCAs
      ii. Bipolar disorder and headaches, particularly migraines—consider treatment with topiramate or valproate
         1. Warn patient about potential weight loss with topiramate.
         2. Warn patient about potential weight gain with valproate.

2.33

HEMORRHOIDS

I. Evaluation
   a. General—submucosal pads of tissue composed of arterial and venous plexuses
   b. Mechanism—associated with chronic straining (e.g., constipation, tenesmus, pregnancy, etc.)
   c. Epidemiology—Approximately 4.4% of the general population
   d. Classification
      i. Internal hemorrhoids—originate above the dentate line
         1. Clinical—typically painless; called to patient's attention if bleeding or prolapsed

    a. Bleeding described as red spotting, usually at the end of defecation.

    b. Prolapse can create a feeling of pressure or mass.

2. Grades

    a. Grade I—bulge with defecation; do not prolapse.

    b. Grade II—prolapse with defecation, but reduces spontaneously.

    c. Grade III—prolapse with defecation and require manual reduction.

    d. Grade IV—prolapse with defecation and cannot be reduced.

ii. External hemorrhoids—originate below the dentate line and covered by anoderm

1. Clinical—associated with discomfort; can be acutely painful if thrombosed.

    a. Bleeding occurs in setting of an automatically resolved local thrombosis.

iii. Mixed hemorrhoids (includes both internal and external)

NOTE:

Patients typically misuse the term *hemorrhoids* to refer to any anal symptoms; make sure to have a complete physical performed to rule out anal fissures, fistulas, abscesses, pruritus ani, condyloma acuminatum, and malignancy.

II. Treatment

  a. Lifestyle changes → goal—to minimize prolonged straining

    i. Increase dietary fiber to 25 to 30 g of fiber per day.

1. Psyllium (Metamucil) 1 to 2 teaspoons in 8 oz of liquid daily to TID

2. Methylcellulose (Citrucel) 1 large tablespoon in 8 oz of cold water daily to TID

    ii. Increase decaffeinated beverages.

  b. Soothing agents

    i. Sitz baths—soaking the anal region in warm water for 15 minutes TID to QID.

    ii. Preparation H cream—apply externally or in lower portion of anal canal up to four times per day.

    iii. Hydrocortisone 1% (preparation H hydrocortisone)—apply to affected area up to four times per day.

NOTE:

Long-term use of any product containing steroids (i.e., hydrocortisone) does increase the risk of a fungal infection.

---

    iv. Preparation H suppository—insert one suppository into the rectum up to four times per day.

Note: Similar products are made under the Tucks brand (formerly Anusol).

  c. Anti-inflammatory medications and analgesics
    i. Most acutely thrombosed external hemorrhoids get better; may just need pain control (through oral medications).
  d. Office-based therapies—rubber-band ligation, infrared photocoagulation, and sclerotherapy
    i. For grade I to III internal hemorrhoids that continue to bleed
  e. Procedure for prolapsing hemorrhoids (PPH) (stapled hemorrhoidectomy)
    i. For grade II to III internal hemorrhoids that have failed rubber-band ligation.
  f. Surgical hemorrhoidectomy
    i. For acutely thrombosed hemorrhoids or grade III to IV internal hemorrhoids

---

2.34

HERPES SIMPLEX VIRUS

I. Evaluation
  a. General—family of viruses responsible for varied infections including
    i. Herpes simplex virus 1 (HSV1)—typically associated with nongenital infections (orofacial, encephalitis)
    ii. HSV2—typically associated with genital infections
  b. Structure—HSV is a double-stranded DNA virus.
  c. Mechanism—to spread, the virus relies on contact between one who is shedding virus and a host.
    i. Contact must be with a mucosal surface or open skin to begin the infectious process.
    ii. The virus can then establish itself in sensory neurons and can be reactivated at a later date.
  d. Epidemiology—most humans have been infected with HSV and maintain latent virus.
  e. Diagnosis—for a definitive diagnosis, isolate the virus from an affected site or bodily fluids.
    i. Can perform a cell culture (PCR) to detect HSV DNA
II. Clinical manifestations
  a. Gingivostomatitis (usually HSV1)
    i. Clinical—fever, sore throat, erythema—vesicular lesions on oral/pharyngeal mucosa

  ii. Risk factors for recurrence—triggers include fever, stress, and so on
    1. Typically found on border of the lip as herpes simplex labialis (cold sores)
b. Herpetic simplex keratitis (usually HSV1)
  i. Clinical—conjunctivitis (most common infectious cause of blindness in the United States)
c. Additional cutaneous manifestations of herpes
  i. Herpetic whitlow—herpetic lesions on open skin or fingers of health care workers
  ii. Herpes gladiatorum—disseminated cutaneous herpetic infection associated with wrestlers
d. Herpes simplex encephalitis (usually HSV1)
  i. Clinical—fever, headache, altered mental status, temporal lobe involvement
  ii. Mechanism—unilateral disease that causes hemorrhagic necrosis of the temporal lobe
  iii. Epidemiology—mortality and morbidity are high even with treatment.
e. Genital herpes (usually HSV2)
  i. Clinical—fever, malaise, inguinal lymphadenopathy → vesicles at primary infection
    1. Recurrence varies greatly from individual to individual.
    2. Complications (aseptic meningitis, urinary retention) are common in women.
  ii. Epidemiology—Twenty percent of Americans have genital herpes; risk factor for human immunodeficiency virus (HIV).

NOTE:

The differential diagnosis for genital herpes includes primary syphilis, chancroid (caused by Haemophilus ducreyi), Crohn's disease, Behçet's syndrome, reactive arthritis, psoriasis, lichen planus, contact dermatitis, and so on.

---

f. Neonatal HSV Infection (usually HSV2)
  i. Clinical—It includes cutaneous lesions, encephalitis, or disseminated infection.
  ii. Mechanism—fetus contacts infected genital secretions from mother at delivery.
  iii. Epidemiology—mortality and morbidity are high, especially for disseminated infection.
III. Herpes simplex virus in the immunocompromised host
  a. General—typically occurs from reactivation of a latent herpes infection
  b. Clinical—includes disseminated cutaneous infection, pneumonitis, gastrointestinal (GI) manifestations, and so on
IV. Treatment
  a. Mucocutaneous

      i. Immunocompromised patients
        1. Acyclovir (Zovirax) 200 to 400 mg PO five times per day
           × 10 days
          OR Valacyclovir (Valtrex) 500 mg PO BID OR 2,000 mg
          q12h × 1 day
          OR Famciclovir (Famvir) 500 mg PO BID × 7 days
      ii. Nonimmunocompromised patients
        1. Acyclovir ointment 5% (Zovirax ointment)—apply six
          times per day × 7 days
   b. Encephalitis
      i. Acyclovir 10 to 15 mg per kg IV q8h × 14 to 21 days
        Note: Keep patient well-hydrated and watch for renal dys-
        function
   c. Genital
      i. Initial episode (shortens symptoms by 2 days)
        1. Acyclovir 200 mg PO five times per day OR 400 mg PO
          TID × 7 to 10 days
          OR Valacyclovir 1,000 mg PO BID × 7 to 10 days
          OR Famciclovir 250 mg TID × 7 to 10 days
      ii. Recurrent episode (shortens symptoms by 1 day)
        1. Acyclovir 200 mg PO five times per day OR 800 mg PO
          BID × 5 days
          OR Valacyclovir 500 mg PO BID × 5 days
          OR Famciclovir 125 mg PO BID × 5 days
      iii. Suppressive therapy (~70% of patients are recurrence-free
        after 4 months)
        1. Acyclovir 400 mg PO BID
          OR Valacyclovir 500 or 1,000 mg PO daily
          OR Famciclovir 250 mg PO BID

2.35

HYPERLIPIDEMIA

I. Evaluation
   a. General—a significant contributor to atherosclerosis and conse-
      quently coronary heart disease (CHD)
      i. Low-density lipoprotein (LDL) is a primary mediator of
        atherosclerosis.
   b. Epidemiology—CHD accounts for 500,000 deaths per year in
      the United States (no.1 cause of morbidity and mortality)

c. Screening—fasting lipid profile (total cholesterol, LDL, high-density lipoprotein [HDL], and triglycerides [TG]) q5yr for patients of age 20 years or older.

REMEMBER:

The lipid profile can NOT be interpreted without knowing the patient's risk factors and CHD risk equivalents.

---

d. Risk factors impacting LDL goals
   i. Age (men of age 45 years or older, women of age 55 years or older)
   ii. HDL <40 mg per dL
   iii. Smoking
   iv. Hypertension (blood pressure [BP] >140/90 or patient is taking antihypertensives)
   v. Family history of premature CHD (first degree male younger than 55 years, first degree female younger than 65 years)

NOTE:

Having a high HDL (>60 mg/dL) is a negative risk factor, and therefore negates having one of the above risk factors.

---

e. CHD risk equivalents
   i. Diabetes
   ii. Framingham risk score (age, cholesterol, HDL, BP, smoking status) of 20% or higher
f. Risk stratification and assessment (see Table 2.35.1)
II. Treatment—may try therapeutic lifestyle changes (TLC) for 12 weeks before considering medications.
   a. TLC
      i. Diet—low in saturated fat and trans fatty acids; cholesterol <200 mg per day
      ii. Physical activity—aerobic exercise increases HDL and decreases TG
      iii. Weight loss—decreases LDL and improves insulin sensitivity

---

TABLE 2.35.1   Risk Assessment for CHD

Risk Category	LDL goal
CHD or CHD risk equivalent	<100 mg/dL
≥2 risk factors	<130 mg/dL
0 or 1 risk factor	<160 mg/dL

CHD, coronary heart disease; LDL, low-density lipoprotein.
Adapted from Executive Summary of the Third Report of the National Cholesterol Education Program (NCEP). Expert panel on detection, evaluation, and treatment of high blood cholesterol in adults (Adult Treatment Panel III). *JAMA.* 2001;285:2486–2487.

iv. No smoking—increases HDL
b. Medications (initially check lipid profile and liver function tests (LFTs) every 6 weeks, then q6mo to every 12 months when LDL is normal)
    i. Statins (↓ LDL significantly, ↑ HDL somewhat, ↓ TG somewhat)
      1. Rosuvastatin (Crestor) 5 to 40 mg PO daily
      2. Atorvastatin (Lipitor) 10 to 80 mg PO daily
      3. Simvastatin (Zocor) 10 to 80 mg PO every evening
      4. Lovastatin (Mevacor) 10 to 80 mg PO every evening
      5. Pravastatin (Pravachol) 10 to 80 mg PO daily
      6. Fluvastatin (Lescol) 20 to 80 mg PO every evening
      Note: Watch for myalgias and rhabdomyolysis with statins.
    ii. Fibric acids (↓ LDL slightly, ↑ HDL, ↓ TG significantly)
      1. Gemfibrozil (Lopid) 600 mg PO BID 30 minutes before meals
      2. Fenofibrate (Tricor) 48 to 145 mg PO daily

NOTE:

Combination of fibric acids and statins increases the risk of myopathy and rhabdomyolysis.

---

    iii. Nicotinic acid (↓ LDL slightly, ↑ HDL significantly, ↓ TG)
      1. Nicotinic acid (niacin) 250 mg to 2 g PO BID to TID
      2. Niaspan (niacin) 500 mg to 2 g PO qhs
      Note: Increase slowly; give aspirin 325 mg 30 minutes before taking niacin to decrease flushing.
    iv. Cholesterol absorption inhibitors (↓ LDL, ↑ HDL, ↓ TG)
      1. Ezetimibe (Zetia) 10 mg PO daily. (Sold in combination with simvastatin as Vytorin)
    v. Bile acid sequestrants (↓ LDL, ↑ HDL minimally, no effect on TG)
      1. Cholestyramine (Questran) 2 to 8 g powder PO BID
      2. Colestipol (Colestid) 2 to 16 g tablets PO divided daily to BID
c. Treatment goals for TG (see Table 2.35.2)
III. Additional considerations—the metabolic syndrome (syndrome X, insulin resistance syndrome)
a. General—associated with insulin resistance and hyperinsulinemia; target after achieving LDL goals
b. Clinical—(three or more of the following are present)
    i. Fasting blood sugar ≥110 mg per dL
    ii. Abdominal obesity (>40 in. waist circumference for men, >35 in. for women)
    iii. TG ≥150 mg per dL
    iv. HDL <40 mg per dL for men, <50 mg per dL for women
    v. BP ≥130/85

TABLE **2.35.2** Treatment Goals for Triglycerides		
Triglyceride Level (mg/dL)	Classification	Treatment
<150	Normal	None indicated
150–199	Borderline-high	Decrease weight; increase physical activity
200–499	High	As above and achieve target non-HDL goal (so, ↓ LDL and TG)
≥500	Very high	As above, but primary goal is to ↓ TG, then ↓ LDL

HDL, high-density lipoprotein; LDL, low-density lipoprotein; TG, triglycerides; ↓, decrease.
Adapted with permission from Executive Summary of the Third Report of the National Cholesterol Education Program (NCEP). Expert panel on detection, evaluation, and treatment of high blood cholesterol in adults (Adult Treatment Panel III). *JAMA.* 2001;285:2486–2487.

    c. Epidemiology—estimated to affect 70 to 80 million people in the United States
    d. Treatment
       i. Lifestyle changes (target obesity, physical inactivity, etc.)
      ii. Treat blood sugar, TGs, HDL, BP, and so on

2.36

HYPERTENSION (ESSENTIAL/PRIMARY)

I. Evaluation
    a. General—essential/primary hypertension is idiopathic and a risk factor for cardiovascular disease.

> **NOTE:**
>
> A 5% to 10% of hypertension is secondary, and therefore due to an identifiable cause; for example, coarctation of the aorta, renal/renovascular disease, alcohol, pregnancy, endocrine (aldosteronism, Cushing's, oral contraceptive pills [OCPs]), and exogenous.

    b. Epidemiology—25% of adults in the United States have hypertension (>140/90 mm Hg).

TABLE 2.36.1 Blood Pressure Classification

Systolic Blood Pressure (mm Hg)	Diastolic Blood Pressure (mm Hg)	Classification
<120	<80	Normal
120–139	80–89	Prehypertension
140–159	90–99	Stage 1
≥160	≥100	Stage 2

On the basis of an average of two or more blood pressure measurements at three or more visits.

(Adapted from Miller ER, Jehn ML. New high blood pressure guidelines create new at-risk classification. *J Cardiovasc Nurs.* 2004;19(6):367–371.)

    c. Risk assessment—risk for cardiovascular disease in hypertensive patients is determined by the following factors:

        i. Level of blood pressure (classification as per Seventh Report of the Joint National Committee) (see Table 2.36.1)

> **NOTE:**
>
> For each increment of 20/10 mm Hg beyond a blood pressure (BP) of 115/75, the risk of cardiovascular disease doubles.

        ii. Major risk factors
1. Smoking
2. Diabetes mellitus (DM)
3. Hyperlipidemia
4. Age older than 60 years
5. Sex (men and postmenopausal women)
6. Family history of cardiovascular disease (men younger than 55 years, women younger than 65 years)

        iii. Target organ damage
1. Heart disease (left ventricular hypertrophy, angina, myocardial infarction [MI], congestive heart failure [CHF])
2. Cerebrovascular disease (stroke, transient ischemic attack)
3. Peripheral arterial disease
4. Nephropathy
5. Retinopathy

    d. Diagnostic algorithm

        i. Routine laboratory tests—urinalysis, complete blood counts (CBC), Chem-7, fasting blood sugar, lipid profile, and electrocardiogram (EKG)

        ii. Lifestyle modification and medication considerations
1. BP 130 to 139/85 to 89
    a. Without DM—modify lifestyle
    b. With DM—modify lifestyle + medication

2. Stage 1 hypertension
    a. No risk factors or target organ disease—modify lifestyle × 1 year, then medications if BP is still ≥140/90
    b. More than one risk factor; no target organ disease—modify lifestyle × 6 months, then medications if BP is still ≥140/90
    c. Target organ disease or DM—modify lifestyle and medication
3. Stage 2 hypertension—modify lifestyle and medication

II. Treatment
  a. Lifestyle modification
    i. Physical activity (30 minutes of aerobic exercise on most days of the week)
    ii. Weight loss (target body mass index [BMI] is 18–24.9)
    iii. Dietary Approaches to Stop Hypertension (DASH) diet
       1. Increase fruits and vegetables, low-fat dairy products, decrease saturated and total fat
    iv. Limit alcohol use (less than two drinks/day for men, less than one drink/day for women)
    v. Limit sodium consumption (<2.4 g/day)
  b. Pharmacotherapy
    i. Diuretics
       1. Indications
          a. First line for uncomplicated hypertension, particularly in older African Americans
          b. CHF
          c. Systolic hypertension
          d. If used as a second-line agent, diuretics can enhance effects of other agents
       2. Contraindications
          a. Gout (diuretics cause hyperuricemia)
       3. Additional side effects
          a. ↓ K (may need to provide patient with potassium supplementation.)
          b. ↓ Na
          c. Glucose intolerance (high-dose diuretic may be unfavorable with DM.)
          d. Hyperlipidemia (high-dose diuretic may be unfavorable with hyperlipidemia.)
          e. ↑ Ca (with *thiazide diuretics*, therefore, may be beneficial in osteoporosis.)
          f. Impotence (with *thiazide diuretics*)
       4. Medications
          a. Thiazide
             i. Hydrochlorothiazide (HCTZ) 12.5 to 50 mg PO daily
             ii. Metolazone (Zaroxolyn) 2.5 to 10 mg PO daily
          b. Loop

        i.   Furosemide (Lasix) 20 to 120 mg PO BID
        ii. Bumetanide (Bumex) 0.5 to 2 mg PO BID
    c. Potassium-sparing: (watch for hyperkalemia; avoid with renal insufficiency)
        i.   Spironolactone (Aldactone) 25 to 100 mg PO daily
        ii. Triamterene (Dyrenium) 25 to 100 mg PO daily
    d. Combination therapy
        i.   HCTZ/triamterene (Maxzide) 25/37.5 or 50/75 mg PO daily

ii. β-Blockers
  1. Indications
    a. First line for uncomplicated hypertension, particularly in young whites
    b. Angina and previous MI
    c. CHF (but avoid β-blockers if patient is having an acute exacerbation)
    d. Tachyarrhythmias (atrial tachycardia, atrial fibrillation, etc.)
    e. Migraine headache
  2. Contraindications
    a. Bronchospastic disease (asthma, chronic obstructive pulmonary disease [COPD])
    b. Second or third degree heart block
  3. Additional side effects
    a. Bradycardia
    b. Heart failure (avoid in acute CHF exacerbation)
    c. Peripheral vascular disease
    d. ↑ Triglycerides (therefore, may have an unfavorable effect on dyslipidemia)
    e. Fatigue, insomnia, decreased exercise tolerance
    f. Depression
  4. Medications
    a. Atenolol (Tenormin) 25 to 100 mg PO daily.
    b. Metoprolol tartrate (Lopressor) 50 to 200 mg PO BID
    c. Metoprolol succinate (Toprol XL) 25 to 400 mg PO daily
    d. Propranolol (Inderal) 40 to 240 mg PO BID
  5. Dual action medications (α_1 blocker and β-blocker)
    a. Carvedilol (Coreg) 3.125 to 25 mg PO BID
    b. Labetalol (Trandate) 200 to 600 mg PO BID (also with IV formulation)

iii. ACE-inhibitors (ACE-Is)
  1. Indications
    a. Previous MI (particularly with systolic dysfunction)
    b. CHF, left ventricular dysfunction
    c. Diabetes or other nephropathy with proteinuria
  2. Contraindications

      a. Pregnancy (teratogen)
      b. Caution with renal insufficiency; avoid in bilateral renal artery stenosis
      c. Hyperkalemia
  3. Additional side effects
      a. Cough
      b. Angioedema
  4. Medications
      a. Captopril (Capoten) 12.5 to 50 mg PO TID
      b. Benazepril (Lotensin) 5 to 40 mg PO daily (may divide BID)
      c. Enalapril (Vasotec) 5 to 40 mg PO daily (may divide BID)
      d. Lisinopril (Prinivil, Zestril) 5 to 40 mg PO daily
      e. Ramipril (Altace) 1.25 to 20 mg PO daily

iv. Angiotensin receptor blockers (ARBs)
  1. Indications
      a. For those patients who cannot tolerate an ACE-I due to cough
      b. CHF
      c. Diabetes or other nephropathy with proteinuria
  2. Contraindications
      a. Pregnancy (teratogen)
      b. Caution with renal insufficiency; avoid in bilateral renal artery stenosis
      c. Hyperkalemia
  3. Additional side effects
      a. angioedema
  4. Medications
      a. Valsartan (Diovan) 80 to 320 mg PO daily
      b. Losartan (Cozaar) 25 to 100 mg PO daily (may divide BID)
      c. Candesartan (Atacand) 8 to 32 mg PO daily (may divide BID)

v. Calcium-channel blockers (CCBs)
  1. Indications
      a. OK for uncomplicated hypertension, particularly in older African Americans
      b. Systolic hypertension (particularly, long-acting dihydropyridines)
      c. Cyclosporine-induced hypertension
      d. Atrial tachycardia, atrial fibrillation (nondihydropyridines)
  2. Contraindications
      a. Second or third degree heart block (nondihydropyridines)

3. Additional side effects
   a. Short-acting CCBs may cause cardiac ischemia by acute hypotension.
   b. Heart failure
   c. Gingival hyperplasia
   d. Edema
   e. Headache
4. Medications
   a. Nondihydropyridines (less potent vasodilators)
      i. Diltiazem (Cardizem) 30 to 90 mg PO QID
         OR Cardizem CD 120 to 480 mg PO daily
      ii. Verapamil (Calan) 80 to 120 mg PO TID
         OR Calan SR 180 to 480 mg PO daily.
   b. Dihydropyridines (greater selectivity for vascular smooth muscle)
      i. Amlodipine (Norvasc) 2.5 to 10 mg PO daily
      ii. Nifedipine SR (Procardia XL) 30 to 120 mg PO daily

vi. α_1-blockers
   1. Indications (not as effective as other medications in decreasing cardiovascular risk)
      a. Prostatic hypertrophy
   2. Contraindications
      a. Orthostatic hypotension
   3. Additional side effects
      a. Headache
      b. Fatigue, weakness
      c. Postural hypotension (so give medication at bedtime)
   4. Medications
      a. Doxazosin (Cardura) 1 to 16 mg PO qhs
      b. Terazosin (Hytrin) 1 to 20 mg PO qhs

vii. Central α_2-agonists
   1. Medications (beware of rebound hypertension)
      a. Clonidine (Catapres) 0.1 to 0.6 mg PO BID
         OR Clonidine transdermal (Catapres-TTS) 0.1 to 0.6 mg per day

viii. Direct acting smooth-muscle vasodilators
   1. Medications (may induce reflex sympathetic stimulation and edema)
      a. Hydralazine 10 to 50 mg PO QID (also with IM/IV formulations)

NOTE:

Patients started on antihypertensive medications should be followed up closely to determine BP control and to monitor for side effects.

III. Hypertensive crises
   a. Hypertensive emergency (typically ≥180/120 and end-organ involvement)
      i. Clinical—requires immediate decrease in BP to minimize or prevent end-organ damage
         1. Malignant hypertension → retinal damage and possible renal involvement
         2. Hypertensive encephalopathy → cerebral edema from hypertension
      ii. Treatment—(lower BP by 25% in first 2 hours, and then toward 160/100 in the next 4 hours)

REMEMBER:

A dramatic decrease in BP can precipitate cardiac, cerebral, and/or renal ischemia.

---

         1. Vasodilators
            a. Nitroprusside (potential for cyanide toxicity limits use)
            b. Nicardipine 5 to 15 mg per hour IV (avoid in CHF)
            c. Enalaprilat 0.625 to 5 mg q6h IV (avoid in acute MI)
            d. Nitroglycerin 0.25 to 0.3 μg/kg/minute IV and titrate upward as needed
            e. Fenoldopam 0.1 to 0.3 μg/kg/minute IV (caution with glaucoma)
         2. Adrenergic inhibitors
            a. Labetalol 20 to 80 mg IV bolus q10min IV up to 300 mg
               OR Labetalol 0.5 to 2 mg per minute IV
   b. Hypertensive urgencies—(typically ≥180/120 and *no* signs of end-organ involvement)
      i. Clinical—situation where it is advantageous to decrease BP in a few hours
      ii. Treatment—may use oral agents as detailed in Section II.
IV. Psychiatric pearls, pointers, and parallels
   a. Substance abuse
      i. Use of certain substances (e.g., cocaine, stimulants) can increase BP.
      ii. Withdrawal from certain substances (e.g., alcohol, benzodiazepines) can increase BP.
   b. Antidepressants and hypertension
      i. Monoamine oxidase inhibitors (MAOIs) when given to a patient eating tyramine-containing foods (e.g., aged cheese, dried meats, soy products, etc.) can produce an adrenergic crisis (hypertension, tachycardia, fever.).
         1. A specific MAOI diet must be followed while taking MAOIs and 2 weeks after discontinuation.

    ii. Serotonin norepinephrine reuptake inhibitors (SNRIs) (particularly venlafaxine) may slightly increase diastolic BP in a dose-dependent manner.

    iii. Serotonin syndrome may involve fluctuations in BP (see Chapter 3.3).

c. Drug–drug interactions involving psychiatric medications and antihypertensive agents

    i. Tricyclic antidepressants (TCAs)

       1. The combination of TCAs and β-blockers can lead to TCA toxicity.

    ii. Selective serotonin reuptake inhibitors (SSRIs)

       1. Fluoxetine decreases β-blocker metabolism, which can cause conduction abnormalities.

       2. Maternal use of SSRIs has been implicated in the development of persistent pulmonary hypertension in newborns.

    iii. Lithium

       1. Thiazides, ACE-Is, and ARBs decrease lithium excretion and can lead to lithium toxicity.

    iv. Antiarrhythmics (e.g., verapamil)

       1. These can interact with SSRIs, TCAs, lithium, and anticonvulsants resulting in neurotoxicity.

2.37

HYPERKALEMIA

I. Evaluation

a. General—serum potassium (K) >5.0 mmol per L

b. Clinical

    i. Often asymptomatic especially when mild.

    ii. Weakness, paralysis, and cardiac abnormalities may occur when severe (K >6.5 mmol/L).

       1. The severity of the presentation parallels the degree of hyperkalemia.

       Therefore, worsening cardiac manifestations are seen on electrocardiogram (EKG) with hyperkalemia and may be rapid:

        a. Mild/moderate hyperkalemia → subtle EKG changes; peaking of T waves

        b. Severe hyperkalemia → prolongation of PR and QRS → loss of P wave and QRS widening

       c. Extreme hyperkalemia → sine wave
                              → ventricular fibrillation

NOTE:

Hyperkalemia in conjunction with EKG changes is a medical emergency.

---

c. Etiology
  i. Reduced renal excretion (the kidney eliminates ~90% of dietary potassium)
    1. Acute oliguric renal failure or chronic renal failure with a glomerular filtration rate (GFR) <15 mL per minute
    2. Mineralocorticoid deficiency
      a. Addison's disease
        i. Psychiatric correlate—Addison's may present with psychiatric symptoms including depression, irritability, psychosis, and cognitive impairment.
      b. Renin and/or aldosterone deficiency
      c. Angiotensin-converting enzyme inhibitors or angiotensin receptor blockers
        i. Work by decreasing aldosterone blood levels.
      d. Nonsteroidal anti-inflammatory drugs (NSAIDS)
    3. Medications that inhibit potassium secretion in the distal nephron
      a. Potassium-sparing diuretics (triamterene, amiloride, spironolactone)
      b. Trimethoprim (TMP) of trimethoprim-sulfamethoxazole (TMP-SMZ)
    4. Type IV renal tubular acidosis (RTA)
  ii. Transcellular shifts (potassium moves from intracellular space to extracellular space)
    1. Acidosis—a decrease in plasma pH of 0.1 causes an increase in serum potassium of 0.6 mmol per L
    2. Hyperosmolality (as occurs in diabetic ketoacidosis or other causes of severe hyperglycemia)
      a. But, in diabetic ketoacidosis osmotic diuresis reduces the level of total body potassium.
    3. Insulin deficiency (insulin helps to bring potassium into cells)
    4. β_2-Blockers (rarely cause clinically significant hyperkalemia alone)
    5. Diseases of cell destruction
      a. Trauma/burns
      b. Rhabdomyolysis
        i. Psychiatric correlate—may occur in intoxicated patients following a blackout.
      c. Hemolysis/lysis of large amounts of tumor cells
  iii. Increased potassium intake (uncommon unless renal excretion of potassium is poor)

1. Beware of salt substitutes that may contain up to 200 mmol per tablespoon of potassium.
2. Can occur if infusion of potassium is too rapid.

iv. Spurious hyperkalemia (sample potassium is high, but plasma potassium is actually normal)

1. Pseudohyperkalemia—hyperkalemia which is due to release of intracellular potassium during phlebotomy.
   a. If suspected, redraw blood sample to get an accurate serum value.
2. Potassium may be released in the sample when thrombocytosis or elevated white blood corpuscles (WBC) is present.
   a. Owing to potassium moving out of platelets and WBCs after clotting has occurred

d. Diagnostic algorithm (in severe hyperkalemia, treat immediately before doing diagnostics)

i. Step 1 → Evaluate the capability of the kidney's response to hyperkalemia.

1. Transtubular Potassium Gradient (TTKG)
   a. TTKG = (urinary K/serum K)/(urinary osmolality/serum osmolality)
      i. If >5, then suspect a nonrenal cause for hyperkalemia.
         1. Therefore, consider transcellular shift or increased potassium intake.
      ii. If <1, then suspect a nonrenal cause for hypokalemia.

ii. Step 2 → If TTKG is between 1 and 5, then establish why the patient has low urinary potassium excretion.

1. Check a serum aldosterone level.
2. Work up primary adrenal failure if warranted.

II. Management

a. Initial management should be governed by EKG changes.

i. Cardiac membrane stabilization

1. Calcium gluconate 5 to 10 mL of a 10% solution IV over 2 to 3 minutes
   a. Repeat after 5 minutes if EKG changes remain.
   b. Use with caution in those on digitalis because digitalis toxicity can occur.

ii. Shift potassium intracellularly

1. Regular insulin 10 units IV with 50 mL of 50% dextrose
2. Aerosolized β_2-agonist
   a. Albuterol 10 to 20 mg in 4 mL of saline by nasal inhalation over 10 minutes
3. Sodium bicarbonate 45 mEq IV over 5 minutes
   a. Use with caution in those with poor renal function because sodium will increase.

iii. Elimination of potassium from the body

1. Cation exchange resins
   a. Sodium polystyrene sulfonate (Kayexalate) 15 g PO q6h p.r.n.
      OR 30 to 60 g retention enema q6h p.r.n.
      i. Use with caution in those with poor renal function as sodium will increase.
2. Loop diuretics (e.g., Lasix)
3. Dialysis

b. After acute treatment of hyperkalemia, correct the underlying cause.
   i. If secondary to a medication effect, then discontinue culprit medications.
   ii. If secondary to a defect in potassium secretion associated with renal failure, then:
      1. Maintain hydration to assure good urine flow.
      2. Loop diuretics (e.g., Lasix)
      3. Maintain dietary restriction of potassium.
      4. Consider oral mineralocorticoids such as fludrocortisone (Florinef acetate).

III. Psychiatric pearls, pointers, and parallels
   a. Digitalis overdose can lead to hyperkalemia
      i. Mechanism of action—digitalis works by inhibiting the Na–K-ATPase pump
      ii. Treatment
         1. Activated charcoal can bind digitalis if ingestion occurred within 8 hours.
         2. Digoxin immune Fab (Digibind)
            a. Side effects of concern include:
               i. Worsened congestive heart failure
               ii. Increased ventricular response in those with atrial fibrillation
               iii. Hypokalemia

REMEMBER:

Look for nonpsychiatric medications when seeing an "overdose" patient.

HYPOKALEMIA

I. Evaluation
   a. General—serum potassium (K) <3.5 mmol/L
   b. Clinical
      i. Often asymptomatic especially when mild (K = 3–3.5 mmol/L).
      ii. Weakness, paralysis, and cardiac abnormalities may occur when severe (K <2.5 mmol/L).
         1. Losses of large amounts of potassium can precipitate rhabdomyolysis and myoglobinuria.
         2. Electrocardiogram (EKG) abnormalities include sagging ST segment, flat T wave, and U wave.
            a. In those on digitalis, hypokalemia can result in a cardiac arrhythmia.
            b. Psychiatric correlate—lithium can also produce flat T waves or inverted T waves.
         3. Hypokalemia is a risk factor for the development of QT prolongation and *torsades de pointes*.

   > **REMEMBER:**
   >
   > Prescribe tricyclic antidepressants and antipsychotics with caution if the patient is hypokalemic or has other risk factors for developing QT prolongation.

      iii. Hypokalemic nephropathy and paralytic ileus can be found in long-standing potassium depletion.
   c. Etiology
      i. Excess renal loss (common cause of hypokalemia)
         1. Diuretic therapy (thiazide or loop diuretics)
         2. Mineralocorticoid excess (hyperaldosteronism, European licorice)
         3. Carbonic anhydrase inhibitors (e.g., acetazolamide)
         4. Osmotic diuresis—increased tubular flow rates, which increase potassium secretion
            a. For example, in diabetic ketoacidosis (DKA) (glucose acts as an osmotic agent) there is total body potassium depletion.
               i. But, recall that hyperosmolality and acidosis cause potassium to shift from cells to plasma; thereby making DKA patients present with hyperkalemia.
         5. Chronic metabolic alkalosis
            a. Contraction alkalosis increases aldosterone, which decreases potassium

6. Antibiotics (penicillin-like antibiotics, gentamicin, amphotericin B)
7. Type I (distal) and type II (proximal) renal tubular acidosis (RTA)

ii. Gastrointestinal (GI) loss (common cause of hypokalemia)
1. Emesis
a. Potassium losses from upper GI are minimal (10 mEq/L); therefore, hypokalemia is the result of potassium losses from secondary hyperaldosteronism and/or bicarbonaturia.
2. Diarrhea (especially secretory diarrhea)—produces significant potassium losses

iii. Transcellular shifts (potassium moves from the extracellular space to intracellular space)
1. Metabolic alkalosis
2. Medications—insulin, β_2-agonists, theophylline, vitamin B_{12}

iv. Magnesium depletion—low magnesium increases renal potassium loss

---

REMEMBER:

Do not overlook magnesium deficiency as a cause of renal potassium loss, especially in alcoholics or malnourished patients.

---

v. Decreased potassium intake (rare cause of hypokalemia)

d. Diagnostic algorithm
i. Step 1—transient versus chronic
1. Transient acute hypokalemia is usually caused by transcellular shifts of potassium.
2. Chronic hypokalemia is usually due to excess renal or GI loss of potassium.
a. Rule out the most common causes (diuretics, diarrhea, and vomiting).

ii. Step 2—is hypokalemia occurring along side hypertension?
1. If blood pressure is high, then consider elevated aldosterone.
2. If blood pressure is normal, then consider increased potassium loss either through kidney or GI.

II. Management
a. Replacement therapy with potassium salts

REMEMBER:

A decrease in plasma potassium concentration of 1 mmol per L is equal to a total body potassium loss of 300 mEq.

---

i. Guidelines
1. Avoid giving more than 200 mEq of potassium daily to replete a potassium deficit.
2. Administer no more than 20 mEq of potassium per hour.

ii. Treatment
1. Oral potassium (preferred method of replacement)
a. Potassium chloride (K-Dur, Klor-Con)
b. Potassium phosphate (Neutra-Phos K)—for those with low potassium and low phosphate
c. Potassium bicarbonate—may be given in metabolic acidosis with hypokalemia
2. IV potassium (for severe hypokalemia, impaired GI, or neuromuscular effects).

III. Psychiatric pearls, pointers, and parallels
a. Patients with eating disorders are susceptible to hypokalemia due to:
i. Induced vomiting
ii. Use of laxatives with subsequent diarrhea
iii. Use of diuretics
b. Patients with alcohol abuse/dependence are susceptible to hypokalemia due to:
i. Poor food intake
ii. Vomiting
iii. Diarrhea

_2.39_

HYPOTHYROIDISM

I. Evaluation
a. General—state of decreased thyroid hormone with varied clinical manifestations
b. Clinical
i. Symptoms—tired, hypersomnia, dry skin, mild weight gain, constipation, cognitive slowing, and so on
ii. Signs—bradycardia, slow speech, pallor, periorbital edema, delayed relaxation of reflexes, and so on
c. Etiology
i. Primary hypothyroidism (thyroid-stimulating hormone [TSH]) $\uparrow$, free T_4 $\downarrow$)—disorder of the thyroid gland
1. Ninety-five percent of hypothyroidism in the United States is a result of primary thyroid failure, including the following:
a. Autoimmune thyroiditis (Hashimoto's)
b. Ablation (surgical, radioiodine, radiation)

2. Other permanent causes
   a. Congenital (1/3,500 live births in the United States)
   b. Infiltrative disorders (e.g., hemochromatosis, amyloidosis, leukemia, etc.)
   c. Iodine deficiency (not found in the United States, but found in third world regions)
3. Transient causes
   a. Subacute thyroiditis (if viral—painful, if postpartum—painless)
   b. Drug induced (amiodarone, lithium, interferon-α, etc.)

ii. Secondary hypothyroidism (TSH ↓, free T_4 ↓)—disorder of the hypothalamic-pituitary axis
   1. Pituitary tumor
   2. Sheehan's syndrome
   3. Cranial/pituitary radiation
   4. Infiltrative disorders
iii. Subclinical hypothyroidism (mild TSH ↑ [5–20 mIU/L], free T_4 normal)
   1. May progress to overt hypothyroidism.

NOTE:

A TSH that is mildly abnormal in an ill patient should be rechecked once the patient has recovered. Also, TSH may be mildly increased in the setting of certain drugs such as dopamine antagonists.

d. Epidemiology—8♀: 1♂; prevalence increases with age
e. Diagnostic algorithm
   i. Check TSH and free T_4 to establish etiology as outlined in the preceding text.
   ii. Magnetic resonance imaging (MRI) of the pituitary is indicated for those patients with secondary hypothyroidism.
   iii. Check antimicrosomal (thyroperoxidase [TPO]) antibodies in subclinical hypothyroidism.
      1. Note—TPO is an enzyme in the thyroid gland.
II. Treatment
   a. Levothyroxine–generic name for synthetic T_4 (Synthroid, Levoxyl)
      i. Average T_4 dose for a normal adult is 1.6 μg/kg/day.
         1. Adults younger than 55 years with no significant medical comorbidities can start on full dose.
         2. Adults of 55 years or older should be treated more conservatively and started at 25 to 50 μg per day.
      ii. Reevaluate the patient's TSH and free T_4 in 6 weeks; goal TSH is 0.5 to 2 mIU per L.
         1. If TSH is still abnormally high, then increase levothyroxine dose by 25 μg.

2. Repeat this process until TSH is at goal/normal.
3. Once normal, TSH can be monitored annually (as long as no change in status).

REMEMBER:

Levothyroxine should be taken on an empty stomach as different foods/supplements (iron, calcium) can inhibit absorption.

III. Additional considerations
    a. Pregnancy (check maternal TSH within 4 weeks of pregnancy.)
       i. Pregnancy increases T_4 requirement by as much as 40%.
          1. Therefore, pregnant women taking levothyroxine may need a higher dose during pregnancy.
    b. Subclinical hypothyroidism
       i. If thyroperoxidase (TPO) antibodies are positive, then the patient is likely to develop overt hypothyroidism.
          1. Therefore, consideration can be given to starting levothyroxine.
    c. Myxedema coma
       i. General—life-threatening complication of hypothyroidism
       ii. Clinical–lethargy or coma, hypothermia, bradycardia, hypotension, delayed relaxation of reflexes
       iii. Etiology–central nervous system depressants, cold weather exposure, sepsis, trauma
       iv. Diagnostic algorithm–TSH, free T_4, complete blood count (CBC), Chem-7, cortisol level, cultures, arterial blood gas, chest x-ray
       v. Treatment (Monitor in intensive care unit [ICU])
          1. Cover patient to limit heat loss
          2. Levothyroxine IV
          3. Hydrocortisone IV until adrenal insufficiency is ruled out
          4. Treat precipitating factors
IV. Psychiatric pearls, pointers, and parallels
    a. Hypothyroidism and depression
       i. Clinical—hypothyroidism can mimic all symptoms of depression.
       ii. Epidemiology
          1. The incidence of depression in hypothyroid patients is higher than in healthy populations.
          2. Chronic and treatment-resistant depression has been associated with overt and subclinical hypothyroidism.
       iii. Correlate—some animal studies show a correlation between hypothyroidism and decreased 5-hydroxy-tryptamine (5-HT) activity.
       iv. Implication for treatment
          1. T_3 (Triiodothyronine, Liothyronine [Cytomel] 12.5–25 μg PO daily)

a. Used as an augmentation agent to treat depression
b. Potential adverse effects of excess T^3 include irritability, diaphoresis, and arrhythmia
   i. Chronic use can interfere with thyroid metabolism.
2. T_4 (Levothyroxine, Synthroid, Levoxyl)—generally not used as an augmentation agent.

b. Hypothyroidism and cognitive abnormalities
   i. Subclinical hypothyroidism is a reversible cause of dementia and cognitive impairment.
   ii. Hypothyroidism can be a cause of delirium; therefore, consider checking a TSH in delirious patients.

c. Hypothyroidism and lithium
   i. Lithium has antithyroid properties as it inhibits secretion of T_3 and T_4.
      1. The resulting hypothyroidism is usually subclinical.
      2. Goiter can occur in up to 50% of patients treated with lithium.

d. Postpartum thyroiditis
   i. Some case reports describe postpartum thyroiditis coexisting with mania and psychosis.
      1. Psychiatric symptoms resolve with treatment of thyroiditis.

e. Congenital hypothyroidism
   i. Clinical—a preventable cause of mental retardation
   ii. Epidemiology—1 in 4,000 newborns
   iii. Diagnostic algorithm—newborns are screened by checking a TSH level.
   iv. Treatment—start thyroxine within 14 days

2.40

INFLUENZA

I. Evaluation
   a. General—a common respiratory infection that afflicts many people throughout the world.
      i. Influenza season = December through March
   b. Clinical—symptoms are typically of sudden onset; mean duration = 7 days (longer in the elderly).
      i. Fever and cough are the best predictors for influenza (vs. the "common cold").

ii. Additional symptoms include headache, sore throat, myalgia, weakness, congestion, and diminished appetite.

NOTE:

5% to 15% of colds are caused by influenza virus.

---

c. Epidemiology—80% to 90% of influenza-associated deaths occur in adults aged 65 years or older.
d. Diagnostic algorithm—rapid diagnostic tests can detect influenza viruses (typically takes 30 minutes).
   i. Viral culture, however, has the best sensitivity, and can provide subtypes and strains.

II. Management
   a. Antiviral agents
      i. Amantadine and rimantadine
         1. Mechanism—block ion channels formed by influenza A's M2 protein
            a. NOT effective against influenza B
         2. Efficacy—decreases length of illness by 1 day in patients treated within the first 2 days of illness
         3. Dosage
            a. Amantadine (Symmetrel) 200 mg PO daily (or divided BID) × 3 to 5 days
            b. Rimantadine (Flumadine) 100 mg PO BID × 3 to 5 days
         4. Adverse effects
            a. Amantadine—central nervous system (CNS) (anxiety, depression, hallucinations, seizures), gastrointestinal (GI)
            b. Rimantadine—GI (less side effects, but more expensive)
      ii. Neuraminidase inhibitors
         1. Mechanism—prevents influenza A or B from penetrating cells.
         2. Efficacy—decreases length of illness by 1 to 1.5 days in those treated within first 2 days of illness.
         3. Dosage
            a. Zanamivir (Relenza)—two inhalations (10 mg) BID × 5 days
            b. Oseltamivir (Tamiflu) 75 mg PO BID × 5 days
         4. Adverse effects
            a. Zanamivir—bronchospasm, reductions in airflow
            b. Oseltamivir—nausea, vomiting (less likely to occur when taken with food)
   b. Symptomatic treatment (see Chapter 2.15)
   c. To prevent contagion, use droplet precaution isolation for those with active Influenza infection.

III. Prevention
   a. Vaccination
      i. Inactivated influenza vaccine
         1. Selection of virus
            a. Determined on an annual basis and targeted toward the influenza strain most likely to cause an epidemic in the succeeding winter.
         2. Who should get the annual influenza vaccine?
            a. Those at high risk for a complication:
               i. Age 50 years or older
               ii. Long-term care facility residents
               iii. Patients with chronic pulmonary disease (including asthma)
               iv. Patients with cardiovascular disease
               v. Patients with chronic metabolic disease and renal dysfunction
               vi. Patients who are immunosuppressed (including human immunodeficiency virus [HIV])
               vii. Those in the second or third trimester of pregnancy during flu season
            b. Those who can transmit influenza to high-risk patients:
               i. Health care workers/providers
               ii. Long-term care facility employees
               iii. Household members (including children) of high-risk patients
         3. Efficacy—on being vaccinated, there is a lower risk of hospitalization and death from any cause.
         4. Adverse effects
            a. 25% report mild soreness at the vaccination site
            b. Contraindicated for those with hypersensitivity to eggs
   b. Antiviral agents
      i. Who should get prophylaxis?
         1. High-risk patients who are unvaccinated
         2. High-risk patients who are vaccinated after the onset of an epidemic (14 days)
            a. It will take approximately 2 weeks for these people to develop an immune response.
         3. High-risk patients when vaccine virus and epidemic virus do *not* match
         4. Individuals with immunodeficiency
         5. Unvaccinated individuals caring for/living with high-risk patients
         6. Long-term facility residents and staff after a facility-wide outbreak ($\geq$14 days)
         7. Those exposed at home
         8. High-risk individuals who are vaccinated (for optimal prophylaxis)

    ii. Dosage
        1. Amantadine 200 mg PO daily (or divided BID)
        2. Rimantadine 100 mg PO BID
        3. Zanamivir—two inhalations (10 mg) daily
        4. Oseltamivir 75 mg PO daily
IV. Complications
    a. Watch for bacterial complications, including pneumonia.

2.41

MENOPAUSE

I. Evaluation
    a. General—menopause is the lasting termination of menstruation.
    b. Etiology—age at menopause is thought to be attributable to genetics.
    c. Epidemiology—mean age of occurrence is 51; therefore, the average woman will live 30 years beyond menopause.
II. Menopausal symptoms and treatment options
    a. Vasomotor symptoms
        i. Clinical—hot flashes ("flushes") (worsen with fatigue/stress), night sweats, insomnia
            1. Usually last 1 to 2 years after menopause, but in some they can last a decade.
        ii. Mechanism—likely due to estrogen withdrawal rather than low estrogen blood levels
        iii. Epidemiology—affect approximately 75% of perimenopausal females
        iv. Treatment options
            1. Hormonal therapy
                a. Systemic estrogen
                b. Progestin alone—medroxyprogesterone (Provera), megestrol (Megace)
            2. Centrally acting agents
                a. Clonidine (Catapres-TTS) patch—0.1 mg per week
                b. Fluoxetine (Prozac) 20 mg PO daily
                c. Venlafaxine (Effexor XR) 75 mg PO daily
    b. Urogenital symptoms
        i. Clinical—vaginal dryness, pruritus, dyspareunia (painful coitus), urethral irritation, and urinary tract infection
        ii. Mechanism—without estrogen, urogenital tissues atrophy; hence, vaginal thinning, and so on

  iii. Treatment options
   1. Hormonal therapy
    a. Systemic estrogen
    b. Topical estrogen—estradiol vaginal (Estrace vaginal), (Premarin vaginal)
     i. Use these creams in low doses—one to three times weekly.
    c. Estradiol vaginal tablet (Vagifem) inserted twice weekly
    d. Estradiol vaginal ring (Estring) inserted q3mo
   2. Vaginal lubricants (use before intercourse as needed for dyspareunia)
    a. Replens, KY Jelly
 c. Psychological symptoms
  i. Clinical—mood swings, depression
  ii. Treatment options—estrogen can improve mood, but treat the underlying depression
III. Hormonal therapy
 a. Systemic estrogen
  i. General—estrogen-only therapy is appropriate for women who do NOT have a uterus.
   1. In women who have a uterus, progestin should be added for 10 to 14 days per month.
    a. Unopposed estrogen greatly increases the risk of endometrial cancer.
   2. Therefore, dosing is as follows:
    a. Estrogen—21 days on, 7 days off (except Premarin which is 25 days on, 5 days off)
    b. Progestin—use for 10 to 14 days per month if the woman has an intact uterus
  ii. Estrogens
   1. Risks
    a. Endometrial cancer (with unopposed estrogen)
    b. Breast cancer (increased risk with long-term [~5 years] estrogen use)
    c. Venous thromboembolism
    d. Heart disease
    e. Stroke
   2. Contraindications
    a. Endometrial cancer
    b. Breast cancer
    c. Thromboembolic disease
    d. Abnormal vaginal bleeding of unknown etiology
    e. History of malignant melanoma
   3. Preparations
    a. Conjugated estrogens (Premarin) 0.3 to 1.25 mg PO daily
    b. Estradiol (Estrace) 1 to 2 mg PO daily

c. Estradiol transdermal (Climara) 1 patch—apply once per week
d. Estradiol transdermal (Alora) 1 patch—apply twice per week

b. Systemic progestin
  i. General—for those patients with a uterus; given in conjunction with estrogen (as in preceding text)
    1. Dosing—administer for 10 to 14 days per month, either at the beginning or mid-cycle
  ii. Progestins
    1. Risks
      a. Bone mineral density loss
      b. Depression
      c. Breast cancer
      d. Venous thromboembolism
      e. Heart disease
      f. Stroke
    2. Preparations
      a. Medroxyprogesterone (Provera) 5 to 10 mg PO daily

IV. Long-term risks after menopause
  a. Cardiovascular disease

NOTE:

Cardiovascular disease is the no.1 cause of death for women.

---

  i. Management
    1. Alter modifiable risk factors (smoking, obesity, lack of exercise.).
    2. Address illnesses that increase the risk of heart disease (diabetes, hypertension, and hyperlipidemia).
  b. Breast cancer
    i. Etiology—hypothesized that extended estrogen exposure increases risk
    ii. Epidemiology—lifetime risk is 12%
    iii. Risk factors—age, early menarche, late menopause, family history, and prior breast disease
      1. Oophorectomy and a term pregnancy before 30 years of age decrease risk.
    iv. Prevention—screening mammography annually for women aged 50 or older
  c. Osteoporosis (see Chapter 2.43)

NAUSEA/VOMITING

I. Evaluation
   a. General—symptoms which range from benign and self-limiting to chronic and life-threatening
   b. Terminology (acute ≤1 month; chronic >1 month)
      i. Nausea—a vague feeling often described as "queasy" by patients.
      ii. Vomiting (emesis)—forceful retrograde release of stomach's contents through the mouth.
      iii. Retching—repeated contractions of the diaphragm, with or without release of stomach's contents.
      iv. Regurgitation—retrograde movement of gastric contents to the oral cavity.
      v. Rumination—regurgitation of food contents into the oral cavity followed by rechewing.
II. Differential diagnosis
   a. Medications—almost any medication can cause nausea including selective serotonin reuptake inhibitors (SSRIs) and serotonin norepinephrine reuptake inhibitors (SNRIs)
   b. Infectious agent—viral (e.g., Norwalk virus, adenovirus), bacterial (food-borne), and so on
   c. Gastrointestinal (GI) disorders—including gastroparesis, small-bowel obstruction, mesenteric ischemia, and so on
   d. Neurologic disorders—including increased intracranial pressure, labyrinthine disorders, migraines, and so on
   e. Psychogenic disorders—mood disorders, eating disorders, anxiety, and so on
   f. Medical conditions—cardiovascular (e.g., acute myocardial infarction), endocrine disorders, pregnancy, and so on
   g. Postoperative nausea/vomiting
   h. Chemotherapy and radiation therapy
   i. Idiopathic causes—cyclic vomiting syndrome ("abdominal migraine")
III. Brief diagnostic algorithm
   a. Initial history
      i. Acute (infectious, emergent, adverse drug reaction, etc.) versus chronic (gastroparesis, etc.)
      ii. Characteristics (projectile, contents of emesis [food particles, bilious, blood], etc.)
      iii. Associated symptoms (fever, diarrhea, abdominal pain, vertigo, neurologic signs, etc.)
   b. Physical examination

      i. Degree of dehydration may vary
          1. Mild—dry mucous membranes and normal vital signs
          2. Severe—orthostatic changes in blood pressure
      ii. Clues—jaundice, abdominal distension/pain/masses, occult blood, neurologic signs, and so on

c. Laboratory evaluation
      i. Complete blood counts (CBC) (infection, anemia from bleeding)
      ii. Electrolytes (metabolic disarray, uremia)
      iii. Pregnancy test (if applicable)
      iv. Further tests—thyroid-stimulating hormone (TSH) (screen for hyperthyroidism), drug screen

d. Additional studies
      i. Abdominal x-ray, computed tomography (CT), barium study, small bowel follow-through, esophagogastroduodenoscopy (EGD), enteroclysis, and so on
      ii. Brain magnetic resonance imaging (MRI) for severe, chronic, and unexplained nausea and vomiting

IV. Treatment

a. Initial management
      i. Identify and correct fluid and electrolyte disturbances.
          1. If patient cannot take fluids orally, then hospitalize for IV hydration with normal saline.
          2. If patient can take fluids orally, then administer 1 to 2 L of fluid per day divided in small amounts.
              a. If liquids are tolerated, advance to dry foods, broth, and so on (1,500 calories/day).
                  i. Avoid creamy, milk-based liquids.
      ii. Address the underlying cause of nausea and vomiting.
      iii. While causes are being addressed, implement antiemetic therapy.
          1. Anticholinergic agents
              a. Meclizine (Antivert) 25 to 50 mg PO daily
                  i. Used for motion sickness and taken 1 hour before travel.
          2. Antihistamines
              a. Diphenhydramine (Benadryl) 25 to 50 mg IM/IV/PO q4h
              b. Hydroxyzine (Atarax, Vistaril) 25 to 100 mg IM/PO q4h
              c. Promethazine (Phenergan) 12.5 to 25 mg IM/IV/PO/PR q4h
                  i. A phenothiazine antihistamine; therefore, extrapyramidal symptoms (EPS) can occur.
          3. Benzamides
              a. Trimethobenzamide (Tigan) 300 mg PO or 200 mg IM/PR q8h
              b. Metoclopramide (Reglan) 5 to 10 mg IM/IV/PO q6h

      i. Prokinetic effects (can be helpful in reflux gastroe-sophageal reflux disease [GERD], gastroparesis)

      ii. Side effects—Extrapyramidal symptoms, fatigue

  4. Phenothiazines

    a. Chlorpromazine (Thorazine) 10 to 25 mg IM/PO/PR q4h

    b. Prochlorperazine (Compazine) 5 to 10 mg IM/IV/PO/PR q6h

  5. Butyrophenones

    a. Haloperidol (Haldol) 0.5 to 5 mg IM/IV/PO q8h

  6. Benzodiazepines

    a. Lorazepam (Ativan) 0.5 to 2.5 mg IM/IV/PO q8h

  7. Corticosteroids

    a. Dexamethasone (Decadron) 4 mg IM/IV/PO q6h

  8. 5-HT_3 serotonin antagonists

    a. Ondansetron (Zofran) 8 mg IM/IV/PO q8h

V. Psychiatric pearls, pointers, and parallels

  a. Psychiatric medications (antidepressants, mood stabilizers) are often implicated in nausea/vomiting.

    i. These symptoms typically subside as one continues to use the medication.

    ii. To limit the side effect of nausea/vomiting initially, start at a low dose and titrate upward.

      1. For example, Effexor XR 37.5 mg PO daily × 1 week, and then 75 mg PO daily thereafter.

  b. Nausea/vomiting can also be a symptom of a somatoform disorder.

    i. Do not confuse hyperemesis gravidarum (intractable nausea/vomiting during pregnancy) for a somatoform disorder.

  c. Benzodiazepines and typical antipsychotics have been used to manage nausea/vomiting, although this is not first line.

    i. These medications may be used in cancer patients with difficult-to-treat nausea/vomiting.

    ii. Beware of extrapyramidal side effects when typical antipsychotics are used to manage nausea/vomiting.

OSTEOPOROSIS (POSTMENOPAUSAL)

I. Evaluation
   a. General—a disease of skeletal weakness ranging from asymptomatic bone loss to fractures
   b. Epidemiology—affects approximately 8 million American women
   c. Risk factors
      i. Elderly, white/Asian, family hx, small body frame, early menopause, prior oophorectomy
      ii. Modifiable—smoking, excess alcohol, lack of exercise, low calcium and vitamin D, low body weight
      iii. Medical comorbidities—hyperthyroidism, hyperparathyroidism, and systemic corticosteroids
   d. Diagnostic algorithm
      i. Low bone mineral density on dual-energy x-ray absorptiometry (DEXA)
      OR fragility fracture regardless of bone mineral density.
   e. Classification (as per the World Health Organization) (see Table 2.43.1)
II. Management
   a. Nonpharmacologic options
      i. Reduce modifiable risk factors (avoid smoking, stop excessive alcohol, exercise, etc.)
      ii. Calcium supplementation (goal: intake 1,200–1,500 mg per day)
         1. Calcium carbonate (Tums) 500 mg BID to TID
         2. Calcium citrate (Citracal) 500 mg BID to TID
      iii. Vitamin D supplementation (deficient when serum 25-OH Vitamin D [25-hydroxyvitamin D] <15 ng/mL)

TABLE 2.43.1 Osteoporosis Classification

Classification	T-score from DEXA
Normal	≥ -1
Osteopenia	< -1 and > -2.5
Osteoporosis	≤ -2.5
Severe osteoporosis	≤ -2.5 + fragility fracture

T-score compares the bone mineral density of the patient to that of a young-normal woman.

DEXA, dual-energy x-ray absorptiometry.

Information from World Health Organization. *Assessment of fracture risk and its application to screening for postmenopausal osteoporosis. Technical report series.* Geneva: WHO; 1994:843.

1. Vitamin D 400 IU PO daily to BID
2. Ergocalciferol (vitamin D_2) 50,000 IU PO weekly
   a. Typically used for approximately 8 weeks to build vitamin D stores.
3. Cholecalciferol (vitamin D_3) 50,000 IU PO weekly (preferred to D_2 when deficient)

b. Pharmacologic options
   i. Antiresorptive agents (block bone resorption by inhibiting osteoclasts)
      1. Bisphosphonates (first-line therapy; most widely used antiresorptive agents)
         a. Mechanism
            i. Increase bone mineral density
            ii. Decrease incidence of hip, vertebral, and nonvertebral fractures
         b. Side effects—esophagitis; minimize risk by taking with water and standing up
         c. Medications
            i. Alendronate (Fosamax) 70 mg PO weekly or 10 mg PO daily
            ii. Risedronate (Actonel) 35 mg PO weekly or 5 mg PO daily
            iii. Ibandronate (Boniva) 150 mg PO monthly or 2.5 mg PO daily
      2. Selective estrogen-receptor modulators
         a. Mechanism
            i. Increase spine bone mineral density
            ii. Decrease vertebral fracture risk; no effect on nonvertebral fractures
         b. Side effects—hot flashes and venous thromboembolism
         c. Medication
            i. Raloxifene (Evista) 60 mg PO daily
               Note: Antiresorptive agents are used for treatment and prevention.
               The prevention dose of alendronate (Fosamax) is 35 mg PO weekly or 5 mg PO daily.
   ii. Anabolic agents (stimulate the formation of new bone through osteoblasts)
      1. Synthetic parathyroid hormone (reserved for severe osteoporosis)
         a. Mechanism
            i. Markedly increase bone mineral density.
            ii. Decrease vertebral and nonvertebral fractures.
         b. Side effects—concern for osteosarcoma (as was seen in rats); hypercalcemia
            i. Therefore, duration of therapy should be ≤2 years.
         c. Medications
            i. Teriparatide (Forteo) 20 μg SC daily

TABLE **2.43.2**	Recommendations for Osteoporosis Treatment	
Classification	**Management**	**Follow-up DEXA**
Normal	Prevention	2–3 yr
Osteopenia	Prevention and/or treatment	1–2 yr
Osteoporosis	Treatment	1 yr

DEXA, dual-energy x-ray absorptiometry.

> Note: Anabolic agents are used for treatment only, and not for prevention.

   c. Recommendations (see Table 2.43.2)

2.44

PAIN

I. Evaluation
   a. General—a subjective experience involving physical, emotional, and cognitive dimensions

---

NOTE:

Greater than half of all patients do NOT receive adequate pain control.

---

   b. Mechanism
      i. Nociceptive pain—receptors triggered by tissue injury
         1. Visceral pain (internal organ pain)
            a. Pain in hollow organs is poorly localized, crampy, and/or colicky.
            b. Pain in solid organs is poorly localized, achy, and/or dull.
         2. Somatic pain—more easily localized, achy, dull, and/or throbbing
      ii. Neuropathic pain—due to pathologic effects on the central or peripheral nervous system
         1. Described as a radiating electric sensation; can also be sharp and burning.
         2. Associated with paresthesias, dysesthesias, hyperalgesia, or allodynia.

REMEMBER:

Neuropathic pain tends to be more difficult to treat than nociceptive pain.

---

c. Classification
   i. Acute—typically follows an injury, but can be *de novo*; usually improves as tissue heals.
   ii. Chronic—pain lasting 3 to 6 months or pain which lasts ≥1 month longer than expected.
d. Assessment
   i. Scales
      1. Numeric rating scale (1–10).
      2. Visual analogue scale (☺ to ☹).
   ii. Frequent reevaluation is key

REMEMBER:

Many factors including culture and gender play a role in how pain is understood and communicated; therefore, it is important to be sensitive to the patient, family, and other caregivers.

II. Management
   a. Pain management as outlined by the World Health Organization (WHO) Analgesic Ladder (Table 2.44.1)
III. Treatment—aim for the lowest possible effective dose to minimize side effects.
   a. Non-Nonsteroidal anti-inflammatory drugs (NSAID) analgesics
      i. Acetaminophen (Tylenol) 325 to 650 mg PO q4h
         1. Maximum dose is 1 g per dose; no more than 4 g per 24 hours.
         2. For those with liver disease, decrease dose as there is a danger for liver toxicity.
   b. NSAIDS
      i. Side effects
         1. Gastrointestinal (GI) ulceration/bleeding
            a. Therefore, consider coadministration with a proton pump inhibitor (PPI).
         2. Potential nephrotoxicity in those with renal disease as well as in the elderly
      ii. Medications
         1. Aspirin 325 to 650 mg PO/PR q4h

TABLE 2.44.1 World Health Organization (WHO) Guidelines for Pain Management

Pain	Treatment Recommendation
Mild	Nonopioids (Acetaminophen/NSAIDs) ± adjuvant agents
Moderate	Nonopioids + weak opioids ± adjuvant agents
Severe	Nonopioids + strong opioids ± adjuvant agents

Some consider a "fourth step" to be interventional approaches to pain management.
Information from Douglass AB. *Section 1—symptomatic care pending diagnosis: pain. Rakel: Conn's current therapy 2006*, 58th ed. WB Saunders; 2006:1–5.

    2. Ibuprofen (Motrin, Advil) 200 to 800 mg PO q6h
    3. Naproxen (Naprosyn, Aleve) 250 to 500 mg PO q8h
    4. Piroxicam (Feldene) 20 mg PO daily
    5. Diclofenac (Voltaren, Cataflam) 50 mg PO q8h
  c. Cyclooxygenase-2 (COX-2) specific inhibitors
    i. Celecoxib (Celebrex) 200 mg PO BID
      1. May have less GI effects than NSAIDS, but be careful with increased cardiovascular risk.
  d. Weak opioids and opioid-like medications
    i. Propoxyphene HCl (Darvon) 65 mg PO q4h = propoxyphene napsylate 100 mg PO q4h
      1. Be careful with continued use as active metabolites accumulate over time.
    ii. Tramadol (Ultram) 50 to 100 mg PO q6h.
      1. May trigger seizures; therefore, avoid in such patients.
  e. Strong opioids
    i. Side effects
      1. Slow GI motility, constipation (most common side effect)

NOTE:

All patients taking an opioid should also receive a bowel regimen including a stool softener and stimulant laxative.

---

      2. Sedation and impaired psychomotor activity
      3. Respiratory depression (the opioid-naive are more susceptible than non-naive)
      4. Pruritus (itching)
      5. Potential for addiction/abuse
    ii. Medications and single-dose equivalencies (Table 2.44.2)

TABLE 2.44.2 Medications and Single-Dose Equivalencies

Medication	Oral Dose	Parenteral (IV/IM) Dose
Morphine	15 mg q4h	5 mg
Hydrocodone	15 mg q4h	N/A
Oxycodone (Roxicodone)	10 mg q4h	N/A
Methadone (Dolophine, Methadose)	10 mg q8h (acute usage)	5 mg
Meperidine (Demerol)	150 mg q3h	37.5 mg
Hydromorphone (Dilaudid)	3.75 mg q4h	0.75 mg
Codeine—used for cough suppression	60 mg q4h (↑↑↑ constipation with ↑ dose)	37.5 mg
Fentanyl	N/A	0.1 mg (or 100 μg)

↑, small increase; ↑↑↑, severe increase.

Adapted from Douglass AB. *Section 1—symptomatic care pending diagnosis: pain.* Rakel: *Conn's current therapy 2006,* 58th ed. WB WB Saunders: 2006:1–5; Max MB. *Chapter 29—pain.* Goldman: *cecil textbook of medicine,* 22nd ed. WB Saunders; 2004:138–145, with additional information from Micromedex, http://www.micromedex.com.

1. Additional notes
   a. Sustained release preparations:
      i. Morphine—MS Contin 15 to 30 mg PO q8h to q12h
         Kadian 20 mg PO q24h (or divided q12h)
      ii. Oxycodone—OxyContin 10 to 160 mg PO q12h
   b. Combination preparations:
      i. Percocet = oxycodone + acetaminophen
      ii. Percodan = oxycodone + aspirin
      iii. Lortab = hydrocodone + acetaminophen
      iv. Vicodin = hydrocodone + acetaminophen
      v. Vicoprofen = hydrocodone + ibuprofen
      vi. Tylenol no.3 = codeine 30 mg + acetaminophen 300 mg
   c. Numerous routes of delivery for varying opioids
      i. IV (including patient controlled analgesia [PCA]), oral, rectal, subcutaneous, transdermal, intrathecal, epidural
         1. IM is generally avoided as it can cause pain itself.
         2. Fentanyl patch (Duragesic) 25 μg/hr—apply q72h.
            a. Equivalent to morphine SR 45 mg per day
   d. Fentanyl and methadone carry the least risk in renal failure patients.
   e. If one opioid ceases to be effective, consider switching opioids.
      i. Incomplete cross-tolerance occurs when switching opioids.
         1. Therefore, the equianalgesic dose should be decreased by 25% to 50%.
   f. Meperidine is contraindicated with monoamine oxidase inhibitor (MAOI) use or within 2 weeks of MAOI use.

REMEMBER:

Naloxone (Narcan) 0.4 to 2 mg IM/IV/SC is an opioid antagonist given to reverse opioid effect. It is used in opioid overdose.

---

   f. Mixed opioid agonist–antagonists
      i. Mechanism—bind to κ opioid receptors for analgesia and antagonize μ-receptor agonists.
         1. This allows for a theoretical decreased risk of respiratory depression (from μ antagonism).
      ii. Side effects
         1. Effects on κ receptor may trigger psychotic symptoms including hallucinations.

2. Blockade of μ receptor may cause opioid withdrawal in those taking μ agonists.
 iii. Medications
  1. Nalbuphine (Nubain) 10 to 20 mg IM/IV/SC q3h
  2. Butorphanol (Stadol) 0.5 to 2 mg IM/IV q3h
   OR Butorphanol nasal (Stadol NS) 1 mg in one nostril q3h
  3. Pentazocine lactate (Talwin) 30 mg IM/IV/SC q3h
   OR Pentazocine/naloxone (Talwin NX) 50/0.5— Take 1 to 2 tabs PO q4h
   a. Oral use only; if injected, naloxone antagonizes pentazocine.
 g. Partial opioid agonists
  i. Mechanism—partial μ receptor agonist; less likely to cause symptoms of psychosis
  ii. Medications
   1. Buprenorphine (Buprenex) 300 μg IM/IV q4h

IV. Additional treatment for neuropathic pain
 a. Anticonvulsants
  i. These medications require gradual dose titration to limit side effects.
  ii. Medications
   1. Gabapentin (Neurontin) 300 to 1,200 mg PO TID
   2. Topiramate (Topamax) 50 to 100 mg PO BID
   3. Carbamazepine (Tegretol) 200 to 600 mg PO BID
   4. Lamotrigine (Lamictal) 25 to 200 mg PO daily
 b. Tricyclic antidepressants (TCAs)—watch for anticholinergic side effects and cardiac arrhythmias.
  i. Imipramine (Tofranil)—start at 25 mg PO qhs; may gradually increase to 75 mg PO qhs
  ii. Amitriptyline (Elavil)—start at 25 mg PO qhs; may gradually increase to 75 mg PO qhs
  iii. Clomipramine (Anafranil)—start at 25 mg PO daily; may gradually increase to 75 mg PO daily
  iv. Trimipramine (Surmontil)—start at 25 mg PO daily; may gradually increase to 75 mg PO daily
  v. Doxepin (Sinequan)—start at 25 mg PO qhs; may gradually increase to 75 mg PO qhs
  vi. Desipramine (Norpramin)—start at 25 mg PO qhs; may gradually increase to 75 mg PO qhs
  vii. Nortriptyline (Pamelor)—start at 10 mg PO daily; may gradually increase to 25 mg PO BID
 c. Topical anesthetics
  i. Lidocaine topical 5% (Lidoderm)—apply up to 3 patches at a time for up to 12 hours per day.
 d. Corticosteroids
  i. In addition to neuropathic pain, can also help to decrease cancer pain (bone, viscera).

V. Muscle relaxants
   a. General—can help in acute musculoskeletal pain; limited role in long-term management
   b. Side effects—sedation, abuse potential
   c. Medications
      i. Carisoprodol (Soma) 350 mg PO TID to QID
      ii. Cyclobenzaprine (Flexeril) 5 to 10 mg PO TID (Maximum is 2–3 weeks)
          1. Not effective for muscle spasm due to cerebral or spine cord disease.
      iii. Baclofen (Kemstro) 5 to 20 mg PO TID to QID
           OR Baclofen intrathecal (Lioresal intrathecal)
           1. Helps flexor spasms and decreases pain and rigidity in those with spinal cord disease.
      iv. Diazepam (Valium) 2 to 10 mg IM/IV/PO BID to QID
          1. Adjunctive therapy for skeletal muscle spasm from upper motor neuron disease.
VI. Other treatment considerations
   a. Physical therapy—prevent maladaptive deconditioning with stretching, exercise, and so on
   b. Psychological treatments—cognitive and behavioral therapies, biofeedback, relaxation training, and so on
   c. Neurosurgical interventions—nerve blocks, spinal infusions (epidural/intrathecal), and so on
   d. Alternative therapy—massage, manipulation, and so on

2.45

PEPTIC ULCER DISEASE

I. Evaluation
   a. General—lesion of the mucous membrane lining the stomach or duodenum
   b. Clinical—epigastric pain (aching, gnawing) that can be intermittent, dyspepsia, with or without nausea/vomiting
      i. Gastric ulcer—pain occurs minutes after eating and can last for hours (until stomach is empty).
      ii. Duodenal ulcer—pain relieved by eating, but may return up to 4 hours later.
   c. Etiology—many factors are associated with peptic ulcer disease (PUD), although these are the most common

    i. Helicobacter pylori infection—acts by inducing mucosal in-
        flammation and cytokine release.
    ii. Nonsteroidal anti-inflammatory drug (NSAID)/aspirin use—
        acts by inhibiting prostaglandin synthesis, which protects mu-
        cosa.
        1. Those who use these agents are also at increased risk of
            complicated ulcers, bleeding, and so on.
  d. Epidemiology—8% to 14% lifetime prevalence with complicat-
      ing ulcer disease occurring with increased age
  e. Risk factors—(independent of *Haemophilus pylori* (*H. pylori*) or
      NSAIDs)
    i. Advanced age (age older than 70 years)
    ii. History of PUD or complicated ulcer disease
    iii. Concomitant warfarin or corticosteroid administration
    iv. Smokers—These individuals having impaired ulcer healing
    v. Alcohol—unclear effect on patients without coexisting liver
        disease
  f. Diagnostic algorithm—typically encompasses the differential of
      dyspepsia (see Chapter 2.24)
    i. Alarm symptoms (gastrointestinal [GI] bleeding, weight loss,
        obstruction, etc.) require evaluation with esophagogastro-
        duodenoscopy (EGD).
    ii. In the absence of alarm symptoms
        1. *H. pylori* infection
            a. "Test and Treat"—*H. pylori* antibody test (enzyme-
                linked immunosorbent assay [ELISA]) and treatment
                if positive
                i. If symptoms persist, then evaluate with EGD.

NOTE:

Fecal antigen testing for *H. pylori* is more accurate than ELISA with a
sensitivity and specificity of 90%.

---

        2. NSAID/aspirin user
            a. Discontinue NSAID/aspirin; consider proton pump
                inhibitor (PPI) trial.
                i. If symptoms persist, then evaluate with EGD.
II. Treatment
  a. *H. pylori*-related PUD
    i. Triple therapy = Two antibiotics × 10 to 14 days + PPI ×
        4 to 8 weeks (80%–90% eradication) (see Table 2.45.1)
  b. NSAID-related PUD
    i. Primary prevention (patient without PUD)
        1. Low risk patient and no aspirin use—continue NSAID
        2. High risk patient—use either NSAID + PPI/misoprostol
            OR replace NSAID

TABLE 2.45.1 Triple Therapy Regimen for *Haemophilus pylori* (*H. pylori*)-related peptic ulcer disease (PUD)

Antibiotic Regimen	Comments
Clarithromycin (Biaxin) 500 mg PO BID + Amoxicillin (Amoxil) 1,000 mg PO BID	First-line therapy as *H. pylori* is most susceptible to this cocktail (*H. pylori* has high rates of resistance to metronidazole.)
Clarithromycin (Biaxin) 500 mg PO BID + Metronidazole (Flagyl) 500 mg PO BID	Use only in patients with a penicillin allergy

Of note, any proton pump inhibitor (PPI) may be used in triple therapy regimens as no difference has been seen amongst them.
Adapted from Saad RJ, Scheiman JM. Diagnosis and management of peptic ulcer disease. *Clin Fam Pract.* 2004;6(3):569–87.

      3. Aspirin use—increases ulcer risk with multiple NSAIDS; may need to add PPI
    ii. Secondary prevention (patient with a history of PUD)
      1. No aspirin use—NSAID (or celecoxib) + PPI/misoprostol
      2. Aspirin use—replace NSAID with celecoxib and add PPI/misoprostol

NOTE:

Given a history of PUD, avoiding NSAIDs/aspirin would be most prudent; however, risks and benefits must be weighed by the treating physician.

III. Complications of peptic ulcer disease
   a. GI hemorrhage (which makes PUD the most common cause of upper GI bleeding)
   b. Perforation—results in an "acute abdomen" (severe abdominal pain, rigidity, absent bowel sounds)
   c. Penetration—ulcer erodes into a local organ (bowel, pancreas, etc.)
   d. Gastric outlet obstruction (occurs in 1%–3% of cases of PUD)

PERIPHERAL ARTERIAL DISEASE

I. Evaluation
   a. General—type of peripheral vascular disease affecting blood vessels outside the heart and brain
   b. Clinical
      i. Claudication—if in the legs, then pain/fatigue with walking which is relieved by rest.
      ii. Limb examination—diminished pulses, hair loss, brittle nails, scaly and dry skin, pallor, ulcer/gangrene.
   c. Mechanism—narrowing of blood vessels inhibits blood flow; usually occurs in legs
   d. Epidemiology—12 million Americans with peripheral arterial disease (PAD)
   e. Risk factors—smoking, diabetes, hypertension, hyperlipidemia, and hyperhomocystinemia, age older than 40 years

---

NOTE:

Smoking is the most important risk factor; cessation significantly decreases disease progression.

---

   f. Diagnostic algorithm
      i. Screen through ankle-brachial index (ABI), which is the ratio of resting systolic blood pressure at the ankle to resting systolic blood pressure at the arm, as determined by use of a blood pressure cuff and Doppler ultrasonography.
         1. ABI 0.91–1.30 = Normal
         2. ABI 0.41–0.90 = Mild-moderate PAD
         3. ABI 0–0.40 = Severe PAD (evidence of advanced ischemia)

REMEMBER:

ABI may better identify PAD than symptoms and/or examination; ABI correlates with exercise capability better than symptoms.

---

      ii. Treadmill test to assess maximal walking distance and pain-free walking distance.
         1. Depending on severity of claudication, consider pharmacologic therapy.

2. If symptoms worsen, then further evaluate (magnetic resonance angiography [MRA], angiography, etc.).
   a. Consider endovascular/surgical intervention

II. Treatment
   a. Nonpharmacological therapy
      i. Risk factor modification of which the most important is smoking cessation.
      ii. Exercise—walking until near-maximal pain for >30 min, three times per week is most effective.
   b. Pharmacologic therapy
      i. Aspirin 81 mg to 325 mg PO daily (with or without Dipyridamole [Persantine])
         1. First choice antiplatelet medication
      ii. Clopidogrel (Plavix) 75 mg PO daily
         1. Secondary prevention of atherosclerotic events in PAD
         2. May be superior to aspirin
      iii. Pentoxifylline (Trental) 400 mg PO TID with meals
         1. May improve walking ability; insufficient information to support widespread use
      iv. Cilostazol (Pletal) 100 mg PO BID
         1. More effective than pentoxifylline; improves pain-free walking distance
         2. Contraindicated in congestive heart failure patients as cilostazol inhibits phosphodiesterase III
         3. Side effects—gastrointestinal (GI) upset, loose stools

2.47

PNEUMONIA (COMMUNITY-ACQUIRED)

I. Evaluation
   a. General—inflammation of the lungs is typically caused by an infectious process.
   b. Clinical—cough, sputum production, shortness of breath, pleuritic chest pain, fatigue, and myalgias.
   c. Etiology (in immunocompetent patients)
      i. Typicals
         1. *Streptococcus pneumoniae* (pneumococcus)—approximately 66% of bacterial pneumonias

        a. Of note, prevalence of drug resistant *S. pneumoniae* is rising and may require intensive care unit (ICU) care.

    2. Haemophilus influenzae

  ii. Atypicals (*Mycoplasma* and *Chlamydia pneumoniae, Legionella*)—approximately 20% to 40% of cases

  iii. Respiratory viruses (influenza, parainfluenza, adenovirus, respiratory syncytial virus [RSV], and coronavirus)

  iv. Anaerobes—typically found in aspiration pneumonia

  v. *Pseudomonas, Staphylococcus aureus*, and gram-negative rods—typically need ICU care

d. Epidemiology—4 million cases of community-acquired pneumonia in the United States per year.

e. Risk factors—smoking is a risk factor for invasive pneumococcal disease.

f. Diagnostic algorithm

  i. First, diagnose pneumonia based on history and physical and chest x-ray showing a pulmonary infiltrate.

  ii. Predictive rules (e.g.,—pneumonia severity index) help establish if hospitalization is needed.

    1. Contraindications to outpatient treatment

      a. Hypoxemia (O_2 saturation <90% or Pao_2 <60 mm Hg on room air)

      b. Hemodynamic instability

      c. Comorbid condition which mandates hospitalization or frail condition

      d. Inability to take oral medications, or no response to oral medications

      e. Unstable psychosocial situation

    2. Factors, which increase risk from low (outpatient) to moderate-high (hospitalize)

      a. Age older than 50

      b. Comorbid condition (cancer, liver disease, renal disease, congestive heart failure [CHF], and so on)

      c. Abnormalities on physical (altered mental status, vital sign abnormalities)

      d. Laboratory abnormalities ($\uparrow$ blood urea nitrogen (BUN), $\uparrow$ glucose, $\downarrow$ Na, $\downarrow$ hematocrit, $\downarrow$ pH)

    3. For further evaluation, obtain gram stain and cultures of blood and sputum

II. Treatment

  a. Empiric therapy options for outpatients

    i. Macrolide

      1. Azithromycin (Z-Pak) 500 mg PO × day 1, and then 250 mg daily (days 2–5)

      OR Azithromycin (Zithromax) 500 mg PO daily × 7 to 10 days

    ii. Tetracycline
      1. Doxycycline (Vibramycin) 100 mg q12h × 10 to 14 days
    iii. Antipneumococcal fluoroquinolone
      1. Levofloxacin (LEVA-pak) 750 mg PO daily × 5 days
        OR Levofloxacin (Levaquin) 500 mg PO daily × 10 to 14 days
      2. Moxifloxacin (Avelox) 400 mg PO daily × 10 to 14 days

  b. Empiric therapy options for general ward inpatients
    i. Third generation Cephalosporin IV initially, and then transition to PO (10—14-day course)
      1. Ceftriaxone (Rocephin) 1 to 2 g IV/IM daily
      2. Cefotaxime (Claforan) 1 to 2 g IV/IM q6h to q8h and Macrolide (e.g., Azithromycin, as in the preceding text, except IV initially, then transition to PO)
    ii. Antipneumococcal fluoroquinolone (IV initially, and then transition to PO [as in the preceding text])
    iii. β-lactam–β-lactamase inhibitor IV initially, and then transition to PO (10- to 14-day course).
      1. Ampicillin-sulbactam (Unasyn) 1.5 to 3 g IV/IM q6h and Macrolide (e.g., Azithromycin, as in preceding text, except IV initially, then transition to PO)

  c. Empiric therapy options for ICU Inpatients (with NO risk for *Pseudomonas aeruginosa*)
    i. Third generation Cephalosporin IV OR β-lactam–β-lactamase inhibitor IV and Antipneumococcal fluoroquinolone IV OR Macrolide IV

  d. Empiric therapy options for ICU inpatients (with risk for *P. aeruginosa*)
    i. Antipseudomonal β-lactam
      1. Piperacillin-tazobactam (Zosyn) 3.375 g IV q6h
      2. Cefepime (Maxipime) 1 to 2 g IV q12h and Aminoglycoside
      3. Gentamicin 1 to 1.7 mg per kg IV/IM q8h (adjust dosing with peaks and troughs) and Antipneumococcal fluoroquinolone IV OR Macrolide IV
    ii. Antipseudomonal β-lactam and Ciprofloxacin (Cipro) 400 mg IV q8h to q12h

---

REMEMBER:

Once cultures and susceptibilities return, antimicrobials can be specifically targeted to the causative agent.

III. Prevention—utilization of vaccination
  a. Children
    i. Pneumococcal conjugate vaccine in infants
      1. Has decreased serious pneumococcal infections and colonization in children.

2. Has decreased the rate of pneumococcal disease in adults perhaps secondary to vaccinated children.

b. Adults

  i. Pneumovax—contains 23 common serotypes of *S. pneumoniae*.

    1. Whom to vaccinate for the first time?

      a. Older than 65 years old

      b. Long-term care facility residents

      c. Patients with diabetes mellitus

      d. Underlying medical illness affecting the heart, lungs, liver, or kidneys

      e. Asplenia (functional or anatomic)

      f. Patients who are immunosuppressed

    2. Whom to revaccinate after 5 years? (only one revaccination needed)

      a. Older than 65 years at the time of first vaccination

      b. Patients with chronic renal disease

      c. Asplenia (functional or anatomic)

      d. Patients who are immunosuppressed

2.48

SINUSITIS (ACUTE BACTERIAL)

I. Evaluation

a. General—inflammation of the paranasal sinuses and nasal mucosa for ≤4 weeks duration

b. Clinical—similar to an upper respiratory viral infection, but bacterial sinusitis is distinguished by the following:

  i. Purulent nasal discharge

  ii. Unilateral maxillary tooth/facial pain (rule out dental abscess) and sinus tenderness

  iii. Symptoms worsen (congestion, cough, headache, malaise, fever, and so on) after 5 to 7 days

---

NOTE:

Viral sinusitis improves within 7 days; therefore, suspect bacterial sinusitis with persistent symptoms for >7 days.

---

c. Etiology (see Table 2.48.1)

TABLE **2.48.1** Etiology of Sinusitis	
General Information	**Likely Microbe**
Community acquired sinusitis	*Streptococcus pneumoniae* or *Haemophilus influenzae*
Nosocomial infections	Gram-negative bacteria
Dental procedures	Anaerobic
Immunocompromised patients	Fungal (especially *Aspergillus* or *Mucor* species)

Most sinusitis is viral; however, acute bacterial sinusitis is a relatively common complication.
Information from Scheid DC, Hamm RM. Acute bacterial rhinosinusitis in adults: Part I.
evaluation. *Am Fam Phys.* 2004;70(9):1685–1692.

    d. Risk factors—anatomic variation, viral infection, allergic rhinitis, smoking, nasal medications, diabetes mellitus, and so on

    e. Imaging—radiographic findings include air-fluid levels, mucus thickening, and opacification

       i. But, radiography (x-ray and/or computed tomography [CT]) and ultrasonography are of little use for routine diagnosis.

II. Management

    a. Symptomatic therapy

       i. Topical decongestants (effective, but limit use to 3 days to avoid rebound congestion)

          1. Oxymetazoline nasal (Afrin) 0.05%—two to three sprays per nostril BID

          2. Phenylephrine nasal (Neo-Synephrine) 0.25%—one to two sprays per nostril q4h

       ii. Oral decongestants

          1. Pseudoephedrine (Sudafed) 60 mg PO q6h OR 120 mg ER PO q12h

---

REMEMBER:

Use decongestants cautiously in those with ischemic heart disease, hypertension, glaucoma, or prostatic hypertrophy.

---

       iii. Topical anticholinergics (possibly effective; helpful in decreasing rhinorrhea)

          1. Ipratropium nasal (Atrovent nasal) 0.06%—two sprays per nostril q6h

       iv. Antihistamines (possibly effective; typically combined with an oral decongestant)

          1. Brompheniramine (Dimetapp) 8 to 12 mg PO q12h

          2. Diphenhydramine (Benadryl) 25 to 50 mg PO q6h

       v. Nasal corticosteroids (possibly effective; work by calming inflammation)

        1. Flonase (fluticasone nasal) 50 μg per spray—two sprays per nostril daily
- vi. Mucolytic agents (possibly effective; works by thinning secretions)
  1. Guaifenesin ER (Mucinex) 600 to 1,200 mg PO q12h
- vii. Moisturization and humidification (no proven benefit in bacterial sinusitis)
  1. Saline spray, nasal irrigation, mist—promote mucociliary clearance.
- b. Antibiotic therapy

NOTE:

Sixty-seven percent of acute bacterial sinusitis resolves without antibiotic therapy.

- i. When to use antibiotics?
  1. For severe symptoms (temperature $>39^{\circ}$ C or $\sim102^{\circ}$ F, periorbital swelling, dental pain, diplopia, etc.)
  2. For mild symptoms lasting >7 days and ≤4 weeks (thereby defining acute sinusitis)
- ii. Which antibiotic to use?
  1. Narrow-spectrum, first-line antibiotics for mild disease
  2. Broader-spectrum, second-line antibiotics for:
     a. Moderate to severe symptoms
     b. Recent antibiotic use (past 6 weeks)
     c. No response to first-line treatment within 3 days
     d. High suspicion of resistant organisms (prevalence $>30\%$ in the area)
- iii. Antibiotics (duration of therapy is typically 7 to 10 days, unless noted)
  1. Narrow-spectrum, first-line agents (non–β-lactam allergic)
     a. Amoxicillin (Amoxil) 500 mg PO q8h OR 875 mg PO q12h
     b. Amoxicillin-clavulanate (Augmentin) 500/125 mg PO q8h
     c. Cefuroxime (Ceftin) 250 to 500 mg PO q12h
  2. Narrow-spectrum, first-line agents (β-lactam allergic)
     a. Doxycycline (Vibramycin) 100 mg PO q12h
     b. Trimethoprim-sulfamethoxazole (TMP-SMZ) (Bactrim DS)—one tablet q12h
     c. Azithromycin (Zithromax) 500 mg PO daily × 3 days
     d. Telithromycin (Ketek) 800 mg PO daily × 5 days
  3. Broader-spectrum, second-line antibiotics (non–β-lactam allergic)
     a. Amoxicillin-clavulanate ER (Augmentin XR) 2,000/125 mg PO q12h.

       b. Ceftriaxone (Rocephin) 1 g IV/IM daily
- 4. Broader-spectrum, second-line antibiotics (β-lactam allergic)
  - a. Levofloxacin (Levaquin) 500 mg PO/IV daily
  - b. Moxifloxacin (Avelox) 400 mg PO/IV daily
- c. Complications and treatment failure
  - i. Culture and/or imaging may be necessary.
  - ii. Refer to otolaryngologist, as nasal endoscopy may be needed.

2.49

SKIN AILMENTS—ACNE VULGARIS

I. Acne vulgaris
- a. General—disease of the pilosebaceous glands
- b. Pathology—increased sebum, hyperkeratinization, accumulation of debris, and *Propionibacterium acnes* colonization
- c. Clinical—occurs in areas with most pilosebaceous glands (face, neck, chest, back, and upper arms.)
  - i. Defined by the presence of comedones; open = "blackheads" and closed = "whiteheads"
- d. Risk factors
  - i. Obstruction (e.g., shirt collars, cosmetics, etc.)
  - ii. Exposures and medications (e.g., steroids, lithium, phenytoin, disulfiram, phenobarbital, etc.)
  - iii. Endocrine disorders (e.g., Cushing's syndrome, polycystic ovarian syndrome, hyperandrogenism, etc.)
- e. Classification
  - i. Mild—few to several papules and pustules; no nodules
  - ii. Moderate—several to many papules and pustules; few to several nodules
  - iii. Severe—many papules, pustules, and nodules

  Note: Inflammatory acne involves the presence of pustules and cysts.
- f. Treatment
  - i. Topical agents

REMEMBER:

For dry or sensitive skin, use creams and lotions; for oily skin, use gels.

---

1. Topical retinoids (for mild acne; prevents obstruction of pilosebaceous glands)
   a. Tretinoin topical (Retin-A)—apply qhs 30 minutes after drying skin.
      i. Adverse effects—thins stratum corneum, pregnancy class C
   b. Adapalene (Differin)—apply 1 hour before bedtime
      i. Adverse effects—pregnancy class C.
   Note: With all retinoids, allow 8 to 12 weeks of treatment for results.
2. Topical antibiotics (for mild to moderate inflammatory acne)
   a. Clindamycin topical (Cleocin T, ClindaMAX)—apply BID.
   b. Erythromycin topical (Akne-Mycin)—apply BID.
3. Benzoyl peroxide (for mild acne; better on papules, but weaker on comedones)
   a. Benzoyl peroxide—apply daily to BID.
   b. Benzoyl peroxide/clindamycin topical (BenzaClin)—apply BID.
   c. Benzoyl peroxide/erythromycin topical (Benzamycin)—apply BID.
4. Azelaic acid (for mild acne; bacteriostatic and keratolytic)
   a. Azelaic acid (Azelex, Finacea)—apply BID to dry skin.
5. Sulfacetamide (for mild acne; bacteriostatic)
   a. Sulfacetamide topical (Klaron)—apply BID.
ii. Systemic agents
1. Oral antibiotics (for moderate to severe inflammatory acne)
   a. Tetracycline 250 mg PO BID to QID
      Doxycycline (Doryx, Vibramycin) 100 mg PO daily to BID
      i. Adverse effects—tooth discoloration, inhibit skeletal growth
   b. Erythromycin stearate (Erythrocin) 250 to 500 mg PO BID
   Note: With oral antibiotics, allow 6 to 8 weeks of treatment for results give for 6 months to decrease likelihood of bacterial resistance.
2. Oral contraceptive pills [OCPs] (adjunct in treating acne in female patients)
   a. Ethinyl estradiol/norgestimate (Ortho-Cyclen)—take one tablet PO daily.
   b. Ethinyl estradiol/ethynodiol (Zovia)—take one tablet PO daily.
3. Isotretinoin (for severe, nodular, inflammatory acne)
   a. Isotretinoin (Accutane) 0.5 to 1 mg/kg/day PO divided BID

i. Adverse effects—teratogen (restricted access), hepatitis, and hypertriglyceridemia
1. Link to depression is controversial.

II. Psychiatric pearls, pointers, and parallels
   a. Patients with body dysmorphic disorder
      i. If the patient appears to have excessive concerns about his skin (or other body parts), or is functionally impaired by his skin ailment (or other perceived defect), then consider body dysmorphic disorder.
   b. Patients with self-injurious behavior
      i. Patients may pick at healthy skin, scabs, or acne and cause further damage to their skin.
      ii. Monitor for signs of infection because topical or systemic antibiotics may be required.
   c. Medication side effects
      i. Lamotrigine (Lamictal), among other medications, is known to have rash as a side effect.
         1. Be sure to warn patients about this, because the rash can lead to Stevens-Johnson syndrome.

2.50

SKIN AILMENTS—CELLULITIS

I. Cellulitis
   a. General—an acute infection of the dermis and subcutaneous tissue marked by inflammation
   b. Clinical—pain, warmth, edema, and poorly demarcated erythema on a portion of skin
      i. A fever and elevated white blood cell (WBC) count may be present.

NOTE:

Track the progression (or regression) of cellulitis by marking the margins of erythema.

---

   c. Etiology—typically caused by *Streptococci* species or *Staphylococcus aureus*
      i. Blood culture is not indicated in routine cases, but warranted when patients have:
         1. Cellulitis superimposed on lymphedema

2. Cellulitis with a likely seawater or fresh-water source of infection
3. High fever and chills suggesting bacteremia
4. Buccal cellulitis (*Haemophilus influenzae*)
5. Periorbital cellulitis (*S. aureus, pneumococcus*, Group A *streptococcus.*)

REMEMBER:

It is important to distinguish periorbital cellulitis from orbital cellulitis because orbital cellulitis is an ocular emergency; complications include visual disturbances, blindness, restricted ocular motility, and cavernous-sinus thrombosis.

---

  d. Risk factors—skin trauma, "skin popping," underlying ulcer/fissure, edema, liposuction, and so on
   i. Psychiatric correlate—infection in unusual areas of the body may be a clue to intravenous drug use.
    1. Beware of endocarditis in intravenous drug users who present with cellulitis.
  e. Imaging—not needed unless concerned about subjacent osteomyelitis, necrotizing fasciitis, and so on
  f. Treatment
   i. Antimicrobial treatment
    1. Typical cellulitis (duration of treatment is usually 7–14 days)
      a. Initial parenteral options: (for worsening disease, compromised host, or fever)
       i. Nafcillin 1 to 1.5 g IV q4h to q6h
       ii. Cefazolin (Ancef) 1 g IV/IM q6h to q8h
       iii. Ceftriaxone (Rocephin) 1 g IV/IM q24h
      b. Subsequent options: (switch as cellulitis improves; often after ~4 days)
       i. Dicloxacillin (Dynapen) 500 mg PO q6h
       ii. Cephalexin (Keflex) 500 mg PO q6h
    2. Methicillin-resistant *S. aureus* (MRSA) cellulitis (duration as in the preceding text)
      a. Initial parenteral options
       i. Vancomycin 10 to 15 mg per kg IV q12h
       ii. Linezolid (Zyvox) 600 mg IV q12h
      b. Subsequent options
       i. Linezolid (Zyvox) 600 mg PO q12h

REMEMBER:

Linezolid (Zyvox) is a weak monoamine oxidase inhibitor (MAOI), and therefore it cannot be used with foods containing tyramine, or pseudoephedrine, because the combination can cause a hypertensive crisis.

---

    3. Limb-threatening diabetic foot ulcer
      a. Causative agents—anaerobes and aerobic gram-negative bacilli
      b. Antimicrobial options
        i. Ampicillin-sulbactam (Unasyn) 3 g IV/IM q6h
        ii. Meropenem (Merrem) 1 g IV q8h
        iii. Clindamycin OR metronidazole + fluoro-quinolone
    4. Exposure to seawater at site of abrasion
      a. Causative agent—*Vibrio vulnificus*
      b. Antimicrobial options
        i. Doxycycline 200 mg IV initially, then 50 to 100 mg IV q12h
        ii. Ciprofloxacin (Cipro) 400 mg IV q12h
    5. Exposure to fresh-water at site of abrasion
      a. Causative agents—*Aeromonas* species
      b. Antimicrobial options
        i. Ciprofloxacin (Cipro) 400 mg IV q12h
        ii. Meropenem (Merrem) 1 g IV q8h
    6. Buccal cellulitis
      a. Causative agent—*H. influenzae*
      b. Antimicrobial options
        i. Ceftriaxone (Rocephin) 1 to 2 g IV/IM q24h
        ii. Meropenem (Merrem) 1 g IV q8h
  ii. Ancillary therapies
    1. Apply cool compresses.
    2. Administer analgesics for pain relief.
    3. Consider tetanus immunization.
    4. Elevation and immobilization of the afflicted extremity to reduce swelling.
    5. For those with peripheral edema, use support stockings to prevent recurrence.
II. Psychiatric pearls, pointers, and parallels
  a. Beware of interactions between antibiotics and methadone.

2.51

SKIN AILMENTS—DERMATITIS

I. Dermatitis—inflammation of the skin
  a. Atopic dermatitis (eczema)
    i. General—inflammation of the skin typically in those with a family history of atopy

ii. Clinical
   1. Acute flares—erythema, pruritus, with or without serous discharge → encrustation, scale
   2. Chronic—lichenification, fibrotic and pigmentary changes; xerosis (dry skin)
iii. Etiology—evidence suggests genetic susceptibility, leads to immune dysregulation (↑ immunoglobulin E [IgE])
iv. Epidemiology—affects approximately 10% of children and approximately 1% of adults
v. Treatment
   1. Hygiene—bathing and use of moisturizers
      a. Bathe with warm water for 5 to 10 minutes once each day.
      b. Use soap only if needed (mild cleansers = Dove, Cetaphil).
      c. After bathing (and before skin is fully dry) apply moisturizer.
         i. Consider application of Eucerin, Aquaphor, mineral oil, or baby oil.
         ii. Apply ointments (most effective) > creams > lotions (least effective).
         iii. Maintaining skin hydration is critical.
      d. Avoid low humidity environments; avoid rapid temperature change.
   2. Sedating antihistamines (decrease pruritus refractory to moisturizers)
      a. Hydroxyzine (Atarax) 25 to 100 mg PO q6h p.r.n.
      b. Diphenhydramine (Benadryl) 25 to 50 mg PO q6h p.r.n.
   3. Tricyclic antidepressants (their antihistaminic properties decrease pruritus)
      a. Doxepin (Sinequan) 10 to 50 mg qhs
   4. Topical corticosteroids (mainstay of therapy)
      a. (Mid potency) Triamcinolone (Kenalog) 0.025%—apply BID to QID.
      b. (Very low) hydrocortisone (Hytone) 1%, 2.5%—apply BID to QID.
   5. Oral corticosteroids (for treatment-resistant disease)
      a. Prednisone 40 to 60 mg daily × 4 days and taper to nil over 2 to 4 weeks
   6. Calcineurin inhibitors (for short-term use because long-term risks are less well known)
      a. (Mild-moderate eczema) pimecrolimus topical (Elidel)—apply BID.
      b. (Moderate-severe eczema) tacrolimus topical (Protopic)—apply BID.
   7. Other
      a. Cyclosporine, methotrexate, azathioprine, mycophenolate mofetil, or ultraviolet (UV) phototherapy

      vi. Complications
1. Secondary infections with *staphylococcal* (*S. aureus*) and *streptococcal* species
   a. Treatment
      i. Keflex 500 to 1,000 mg PO q6h
2. Eczema herpeticum (herpes simplex virus [HSV] infection)
   a. General—vesicles, crusts, and so on complicating atopic dermatitis
   b. Treatment
      i. Acyclovir 200 mg PO five times per day OR 10 mg per kg IV q8h

b. Contact dermatitis
    i. General—inflammation of the skin secondary to direct interaction of skin with an irritant
    ii. Clinical—eczematous (erythema, pruritus, with or without serous discharge → encrustation, scale)
      1. Varying degrees of edema, vesiculation, and lichenification (hardening)
    iii. Classification
      1. Irritant contact dermatitis (75%–80% of contact dermatitis)
        a. Etiology—exposure to a substance that irritates the skin
          i. Epidermal barrier is broken and secondary inflammation occurs.
        b. Triggers—acids/alkalis such as solvents, detergents, cleansers, and so on
          i. May occur on first contact (burn) or after multiple exposures.
        c. Epidemiology—can occur in anyone; patients with atopy are more susceptible
        d. Treatment
          i. Stop exposure; lavage with copious amounts of water
          ii. Analgesia for pain control
          iii. Wound care (nonadherent dressing; may need debridement)
          iv. Very high or mid-strength topical corticosteroid ointment
            1. Betamethasone dipropionate—apply daily to BID.
            2. Triamcinolone (Kenalog) 0.025%—apply BID to QID.
      2. Allergic contact dermatitis (20%–25% of contact dermatitis)
        a. Etiology—immunologic reaction (type IV) to an allergen on the skin

  b. Triggers—poison ivy, poison oak, nickel, perfumes, chemicals, and so on
  c. Treatment
    i. Avoid the exposure
    ii. Thin wet dressings (tap water, saline, or aluminum acetate)
    iii. Sedating antihistamines (decrease pruritus)
      1. Hydroxyzine (Atarax) 25 to 100 mg PO q6h p.r.n.
      2. Diphenhydramine (Benadryl) 25 to 50 mg PO q6h p.r.n.
    iv. Ultra highpotent topical corticosteroids (2 weeks only)
      1. Clobetasol (Temovate) 0.05%—apply BID.
      2. Halobetasol (Ultravate) 0.05%—apply daily to BID.
    v. Oral corticosteroids
      1. Prednisone 1 mg/kg/day × 1 week, then half × 1 week
    vi. Calcineurin inhibitors
      1. Pimecrolimus topical (Elidel)—apply BID.
      2. Tacrolimus topical (Protopic)—apply BID.
    vii. Other
      1. Cyclosporine, methotrexate, azathioprine, mycophenolate mofetil
c. Seborrheic dermatitis
  i. General—excessive discharge from sebaceous glands (numerous on face and trunk)
  ii. Clinical—"oily" secretion varying from dandruff to dense, adherent, greasy scale
    1. Pinkish erythema and mild epidermal hyperproliferation (scale); mild pruritus
  iii. Etiology—evidence suggests an inflammatory reaction to yeast from the *Malassezia* genus
  iv. Epidemiology—♂ > ♀; 3% of the general population and in AIDS (acquired immunodeficiency syndrome) patients as high as 85%
  v. Risk factors—neonates and those in the postpuberty phase (perhaps from hormonal control [androgens])
  vi. Treatment
    1. General
      a. Hygiene—washing with soap removes oils and thereby improves seborrhea.
    2. Seborrheic dermatitis of the scalp and beard (dandruff)
      a. Antidandruff shampoos—apply and leave in place for 10 minutes prerinsing.
        i. Selenium sulfide 1% (Selsun Blue) or 2.5% (Selsun, Exsel)

        ii. Pyrithione zinc 1% (Head and Shoulders) or 2% (DHS Zinc)

    b. Antifungal shampoo—decrease colonization by lipophilic yeast.

        i. Ketoconazole (Nizoral)—apply daily as needed.

    c. Coal tar preparations

        i. Neutrogena T/Gel, DHS Tar, Denorex, and so on

3. Seborrheic dermatitis in nonscalp regions

    a. Topical corticosteroids (multiple preparations—creams, lotions, etc.)

        i. Desonide (Tridesilon) 0.05%—apply BID to TID.

        ii. Hydrocortisone 0.5%, 1%, or 2.5%—apply BID to QID.

    b. Topical antifungals

        i. Miconazole cream (Monistat) 2%—apply daily.

        ii. Clotrimazole cream (Lotrimin) 1%—apply daily.

        iii. Ketoconazole cream (Nizoral) 2%—apply daily.

    c. Other (i.e., acne preparations)

        i. Sulfacetamide topical (Klaron) 10%—apply BID.

        ii. Benzoyl peroxide (Benzac AC) 2% to 10%—apply daily to BID.

        iii. Isotretinoin (Accutane) 0.5 to 1 mg/kg/day PO divided BID.

            1. Accutane is for treatment-resistant patients only.

  d. Intertrigo

    i. General—skin condition caused by the adverse effect of friction, heat, and moisture

    ii. Clinical—symmetrical erythema typically in body folds with pruritus, stinging, and burning

        1. In severe cases, erosion and denudation can occur.

    iii. Complications—candidiasis

    iv. Treatment—(typically requires 1–3 weeks of treatment; recurrence is common)

        1. General

            a. Maintain hygiene in the affected area; keep area dry.

            b. In the acute setting, compresses can be used.

        2. Topical corticosteroids

            a. Triamcinolone acetonide (Kenalog) 0.025%—apply daily to QID.

            b. Hydrocortisone 0.5%, 1%, or 2.5%—apply BID to QID.

        3. Topical antifungals

            a. Nystatin topical (Mycostatin)—apply BID to TID.

        4. Combination topical corticosteroids and antifungals

            a. Nystatin/triamcinolone topical (Mycolog-II)—apply BID.

II. Topical corticosteroids

TABLE 2.51.1	Topical Corticosteroids	
Class (Potency)	Example Drug	May Be Used to Treat
I (ultra high)	Clobetasol (Temovate) 0.05%—apply BID Halobetasol (Ultravate) 0.05%—apply daily to BID	Allergic contact dermatitis (e.g., severe poison ivy)
II (very high)	Triamcinolone acetonide (Aristocort A) 0.5%—apply daily to BID Betamethasone dipropionate (Diprosone) 0.05%—apply daily to BID	Resistant atopic dermatitis Severe hand eczema Psoriasis
III (high)	Triamcinolone acetonide (Aristocort A/Kenalog) 0.1%—apply daily to QID Betamethasone valerate (Valisone) 0.1%—apply daily to BID	Atopic dermatitis Seborrheic dermatitis Severe intertrigo (short course) Tinea (short course for control of inflammation)
IV (mid)	Triamcinolone acetonide (Aristocort A/Kenalog) 0.025%—apply daily to QID Betamethasone valerate (Valisone) 0.01%—apply daily to BID	Scabies (use after scabicide)
V (low)	Desonide (Tridesilon/DesOwen) 0.05%—apply BID to TID	
VI (very low)	Hydrocortisone (Hytone) 1%, 2.5%—apply BID to QID	Dermatitis (and mild facial dermatitis) Mild intertrigo

Adapted from Goldstein B, ed. *Practical dermatology*, 2nd ed. St. Louis: Mosby; 1997 and Habif TP. *Chapter 2—topical therapy and topical corticosteroids. Habif: clinical dermatology*, 4th ed. St. Louis: Mosby; 2004:23–40.

a. Potency (see Table 2.51.1)
b. Duration of treatment
   i. Class I—2 weeks of treatment followed by 1 week of rest until lesions cleared
   ii. Classes II to VI—2 to 6 weeks of treatment
c. Vehicle (= base)
   i. Creams—greasy, high versatility, most useful for intertriginous areas.
   ii. Ointments—greasy, lubricating, enhanced potency, too occlusive for intertriginous areas.
   iii. Gels—greaseless, good for acute exudative lesions (e.g., poison ivy).
   iv. Solutions and lotions—good for scalp because of easy penetration through hair.
   v. Foams—typically deliver superpotent agents, useful for scalp dermatoses.

SKIN
AILMENTS—ECTOPARASITES

I. Pediculosis (lice)
   a. General—arthropod and obligate parasite which infests humans
   b. Clinical—an allergic reaction to louse saliva produces pruritus; takes ≥2 weeks to develop
   c. Etiology—lice species affecting humans include
      i. *Pediculus humanus capitis*—head louse
      ii. *Phthirus pubis*—pubic louse (crab)
      iii. *Pediculus humanus corpus*—body louse
   d. Transmission—person-to-person contact
   e. Life cycle—egg firmly on hair shaft → nymph after approximately 7 days → mature after approximately 10 days
   f. Risk factors—bedding/clothing changed infrequently, homeless
   g. Diagnosis—lice or nits (viable eggs) seen on examination; excoriation may also exist
   h. Treatment
      i. *Pediculus humanus capitis*—head louse

REMEMBER:

Two courses of treatment are typically needed because developing embryos can survive the first course; therefore, reapply treatment in 10 days, especially if live lice are found.

---

   1. *Pyrethrum Insecticides* (pyrethroids)
      a. Permethrin topical (Nix) 1% cream q10d × two applications
         i. Use after shampooing, leave in place for 10 minutes, rinse.
      b. Pyrethrin topical (Rid) 0.33% foam q10d × two applications
         i. Apply to dry hair, leave in place for 10 minutes, rinse.
   2. Second-line agents for treatment-resistant head lice
      a. Malathion topical (Ovide) 0.5% q10d × two applications
         i. Apply to dry hair, leave in place for approximately 10 hours, rinse.
      b. Lindane topical 1% shampoo × one application
         i. Used infrequently because of neurotoxicity.
   3. Oral agents

   a. Ivermectin (Stromectol) 200 μg per kg PO q10d ×
    two doses
     i. Not indicated by U.S. Food and Drug Administra-
      tion (FDA) for pediculosis.
  ii. *Phthirus pubis*— pubic louse (crab)
   1. Treat as with head louse and evaluate for other common
    sexually transmitted diseases.
  iii. *Pediculus humanus corpus*— body louse
   1. Wash entire body extensively and don clean clothing.
   2. Treat whole body using agents as described in the pre-
    ceding text.

NOTE:

Body lice (as opposed to head lice and pubic lice) may transmit systemic diseases such as typhus and trench fever.

---

 i. Contacts and prevention
  i. Screen all household contacts (or sexual contacts in the case
   of pubic louse).
  ii. Treat those who are infested or who share the same bed (this
   decreases likelihood of reinfestation).
  iii. Decontaminate bedding and clothing—wash in 60°C water
   and use heated drying.
  iv. Decontaminate brushes, combs, and so on—soak in 60°C
   water × 10 minutes.

II. Scabies
 a. General—obligate parasitic mite that affects humans
 b. Clinical—a delayed hypersensitivity reaction to mites, eggs, and
  fecal pellets yields pruritus
  i. A papular rash with excoriations is present; head and neck
   typically not effected.
 c. Etiology—Sarcoptes scabiei
 d. Transmission—person-to-person contact
 e. Life cycle— ♀ mite burrows under skin → eggs hatch after 3 days
  → mature after approximately 2 weeks
 f. Risk factors—household or sexual contacts
 g. Diagnosis—mites seen on examination of skin scrapings (edge
  of the burrow, under fingernails)
 h. Treatment
  i. *Pyrethrum Insecticides* (pyrethroids)
   1. Permethrin topical (Elimite) 5% cream × 1 (re-treat only
    if new lesions)
    a. Apply from head to toe, leave in place for 8 to
     14 hours, wash off.
  ii. Crotamiton
   1. Crotamiton topical (Eurax) 10% cream, lotion q24h ×
    two applications

a. Apply from chin to toe, leave in place for 24 hours, wash, and repeat.
iii. Oral agents (typically for crusted scabies because penetration of topicals can be hard)
1. Ivermectin (Stromectol) 200 μg per kg PO × 1 (timing of second dose varies)

NOTE:

Pruritus may last for approximately 1 month after successful treatment of scabies; manage itching with antihistamines, with or without midpotency topical corticosteroid (but use steroid only after completion of primary scabies treatment).

---

i. Contacts and prevention
   i. Screen all household and sexual contacts.
   ii. Treat those who have symptoms; contacts should also employ cleansing procedures as below.
   iii. Decontaminate bedding and clothing—wash in 60°C water and use heated drying.
   iv. Decontaminate all other items—soak in 60°C water or dry clean.
j. Complications
   i. Secondary pyoderma requires treatment with topical and/or systemic antibiotics.

2.53

SKIN AILMENTS—PRURITUS

I. Pruritus (itching)
   a. General—clinical finding that can result from a dermatologic disease or a systemic condition.
   b. Mechanism—can be due to release of histamine or serotonin, neuropathy, immune based, medications, and so on.
   c. Diagnostic algorithm
      i. Get history and physical examination.
      ii. If typical skin findings, then treat accordingly; if atypical, consider biopsy and/or scraping; if no skin findings, then initiate empiric therapy with skin hygiene and oral antihistamines.
      iii. If treatment is not effective (and/or diagnosis is unclear), then evaluate further.

1. First-tier studies—complete blood count (CBC), thyroid-stimulating hormone (TSH), liver function tests (LFTs), blood urea nitrogen (BUN)/creatinine
2. Second-tier studies—(as applicable) malignancy workup, bone marrow biopsy, human immunodeficiency virus (HIV), and so on

d. Classification
   i. Dermatologic causes
      1. Urticaria (hives)—transient condition mediated by histamine
      2. Dermatitis (see Chapter 2.51.)
      3. Psoriasis—silvery scaly patches
      4. Ectoparasites (see Chapter 2.52.)
   ii. Systemic causes (10%–50% of those with generalized pruritus have a systemic etiology.)
      1. Medication (e.g., opioids)
      2. Thyroid disease (either hypothyroidism or hyperthyroidism)
      3. Infection (e.g., HIV, parasite)
      4. Uremia
      5. Liver disease
      6. Malignancy (e.g., Hodgkin's disease, multiple myeloma.)

e. Treatment
   i. Treat on the basis of diagnosis; therefore, it is critical to identify underlying cause.
   ii. Skin care
      1. Eliminate triggers.
         a. Use fragrance-free soaps and detergents; avoid perfumes, colognes, and so on.
      2. Apply lubricant/moisturizer.
         a. For dry (xerosis), scaly skin with pruritus:
            i. Ammonium lactate topical (Lac-Hydrin) 12%—apply BID.
               1. May cause transient stinging; may irritate face.
               2. Protect areas with clothing when out in the sun.
         b. Frequent lubricating is encouraged, especially after bathing.
      3. Use lukewarm water; avoid hot water.
   iii. Oral antihistamines
      1. First-generation H_1 antihistamines (mainstay medication; sedating and anxiolytic)
         a. Hydroxyzine (Atarax, Vistaril) 25 to 100 mg PO q6h p.r.n.
         b. Diphenhydramine (Benadryl) 25 to 50 mg PO q6h p.r.n.
         c. Cyproheptadine (Periactin) 4 mg PO TID p.r.n.

        d. Doxepin (Sinequan) 10 to 25 mg PO at bedtime p.r.n.
  2. Second-generation H_1 antihistamines (do not cross the blood–brain barrier)
     a. Fexofenadine (Allegra) 180 mg PO daily
     b. Cetirizine (Zyrtec) 5 to 10 mg PO daily
     c. Loratadine (Claritin) 10 mg PO daily
     d. Desloratadine (Clarinex) 5 mg PO daily
  iv. Treatment modalities for recalcitrant pruritus (again, look for underlying cause)
      1. Oral steroids
         a. Prednisone 10 to 40 mg PO daily with taper
      2. Phototherapy
      3. Systemic immunosuppression

2.54

SKIN AILMENTS—TINEA

I. Fungal disease affecting the skin
  a. General—superficial infection of keratin-containing tissues including skin, nails, and hair shafts
  b. Etiology
     i. Dermatophytes (*Trichophyton, Microsporum, Epidermophyton*) = tinea
     ii. Yeast (*Candida*) (see Chapter 2.12)
     iii. *Malassezia* species (e.g., *Tinea versicolor*)
II. Dermatophytes (tinea)
  a. General—consist of spores and hyphae that afflict soft keratin of the skin in different body locals.
  b. Epidemiology—10% to 20% lifetime risk of acquiring a tinea infection.

REMEMBER:

Tinea is the second most frequently reported skin disease next to acne.

---

  c. Diagnostic evaluation
     i. A 20% potassium hydroxide (KOH) preparation is used to visualize hyphae.
        1. Obtain sample by scraping lesion with a no. 15 blade scalpel or the edge of a slide.

    ii. Culture is rarely indicated, although it may help direct oral therapy.

    iii. Biopsy with periodic acid-Schiff stain when the diagnosis remains in question.

d. Classification and treatment

    i. Tinea pedis (athlete's foot)

      1. General—most common fungal infection of the skin

      2. Clinical—erythematous scaling plaques, pruritic, presents as

        a. Maceration between the toes (toe-web distribution)

        b. Diffuse erythema affecting the soles (moccasin distribution)

      3. Etiology—most commonly caused by the dermatophytes *Trichophyton rubrum* and *Trichophyton mentagrophytes*

      4. Risk factors—occlusive footwear

      5. Treatment

        a. Topical—apply medication to include skin approximately 2 cm beyond the affected area.

          i. Butenafine (Mentax, Lotrimin Ultra)—apply daily × 4 weeks.
OR Butenafine (Mentax, Lotrimin Ultra)—apply BID × 1 week.

          ii. Azole—clotrimazole (Lotrimin AF, Mycelex) 1%—apply BID up to 4 weeks.

          iii. Tolnaftate (Tinactin) 1%—apply BID up to 4 to 6 weeks.

          iv. Naftifine (Naftin) 1% cream daily for up to 4 weeks.

      6. Combination topical treatment

        a. Betamethasone/clotrimazole (Lotrisone) 0.05%/1% cream—apply BID up to 4 weeks.

      7. Systemic treatment

        a. Allylamine—terbinafine (Lamisil) 250 mg PO daily × 2 weeks

        b. Triazole—itraconazole (Sporanox) 200 mg PO BID × 2 weeks

          i. Adverse effect—reversible hepatitis, so watch liver function tests (LFTs).

      8. Prevention

        a. Use foot powder that absorbs moisture.

        b. Frequently change socks and shoes (do not allow to become moist.).

NOTE:

As tinea pedis affects the foot, tinea manuum affects the hand.

---

    ii. Tinea corporis

      1. General—tinea infection of the trunk or extremities

    2. Clinical—ringworm (ringed plaque with raised border); later has central clearing

    3. Etiology—commonly caused by *T. rubrum*

    4. Topical treatment

      a. Azole → clotrimazole (Lotrimin, Mycelex) 1%— apply BID × 2 to 4 weeks.

      b. Allylamine → terbinafine (Lamisil AT) 1%—apply BID × 2 to 4 weeks.

    5. Systemic treatment (for extensive skin involvement)

      a. Triazole—itraconazole (Sporanox) 200 mg PO daily × 2 weeks

iii. Tinea cruris (jock itch)

    1. General—tinea infection of the groin; a location of increased sweating and friction

    2. Clinical—pruritic, red plaques on the medial thighs sparing the penis and scrotum

---

REMEMBER:

Candidiasis typically does NOT spare the penis and scrotum when affecting the groin area.

---

    3. Etiology—*T. rubrum, T. mentagrophytes, Epidermophyton floccosum*

    4. Topical treatment

      a. Azole → clotrimazole (Lotrimin, Mycelex) 1%— apply BID × 2 to 4 weeks.

NOTE:

Topical agents do not penetrate hair or nails; therefore, systemic treatments are solely utilized for these tinea infections.

---

iv. Tinea capitis

    1. General—tinea infection of the scalp

    2. Clinical—patchy hair loss and scaling; may have cervical lymphadenopathy

    3. Etiology—*Trichophyton tonsurans*

    4. Systemic treatment

      a. Griseofulvin microsize (Grifulvin V) 500 mg PO daily × 4 to 6 weeks

      Note: Fat aids in the absorption of griseofulvin, so take with meals.

v. Tinea barbae

    1. General—tinea infection of the beard and mustache areas

    2. Clinical—usually unilateral and spares the lip

3. Etiology—*T. mentagrophytes* and rarely *Trichophyton verrucosum*
4. Systemic treatment
   a. Griseofulvin ultramicrosize (Gris-PEG) 375 mg PO daily × 2 to 4 weeks
   vi. Tinea unguium (a subset of the onychomycoses, of which yeast is also a member)
      1. General—tinea infection of the nail plate (toenails or fingernails).
      2. Clinical—nail is thick, brittle, hard, and discolored (yellow/brown); often associated with tinea pedis.
      3. Etiology—*T. rubrum*, accounts for 80% of all nail fungal infections; *T. mentagrophytes*.
      4. Epidemiology—affects approximately 2% of the US population.
      5. Treatment
         a. Topical
            i. Miconazole topical 2% powder applied BID over nail plate
            ii. Clotrimazole topical 1% cream applied BID
            iii. Ciclopirox (Penlac Nail Lacquer) 8%—apply to nail qhs (maximum 48 weeks)
         b. Oral (use these medications with caution, monitor LFTs, avoid with pregnancy, etc.)
            i. Itraconazole (Sporanox) 200 mg PO daily × 3 months
            ii. Terbinafine (Lamisil) 250 mg PO daily × 6 weeks (fingernails)
               Terbinafine (Lamisil) 250 mg PO daily × 12 weeks (toenails).
            iii. Fluconazole (Diflucan) 150 to 300 mg weekly until infection clears

III. Tinea versicolor (caused by *Malassezia* species and therefore NOT a true tinea infection)
   a. General—excessive colonization of a normal skin fungus leads to this ailment.
   b. Clinical—asymptomatic, circular, pink, scaling macules on the trunk; can become confluent.
      i. Can be confused for vitiligo
   c. Etiology—*Malassezia furfur* (formerly referred to as *Pityrosporum orbiculare* and *Pityrosporum ovale*)
   d. Diagnostic evaluation—KOH preparation shows "spaghetti and meatballs" of hyphae and spores.
   e. Topical treatment
      i. Azole—clotrimazole (Lotrimin, Mycelex) 1%—apply BID × 4 weeks.

      ii. Tolnaftate (Tinactin) 1%—apply BID × 4 to 6 weeks.

      iii. Selenium sulfide (Selsun) 2.5% lotion—apply daily for 10 minutes, then rinse × 1 week.

  f. Systemic treatment

      i. Triazole—itraconazole (Sporanox) 200 mg PO daily × 1 week

2.55

STYE (HORDEOLUM)

I. Evaluation
   a. General—acute inflammatory process involving the glands (meibomian or Zeis) of the eyelid.
   b. Clinical—abrupt onset of a tender, erythematous mass of the eyelid.
   c. Etiology—*Staphylococcus aureus* is responsible for 75% to 95% of cases.

II. Treatment
   a. Standard cases
      i. Warm compresses to closed eye QID × 3 to 4 days.
      ii. Erythromycin ophthalmic 0.5% ointment—apply to lid margins BID to QID until resolved.
   b. Refractory cases
      i. Oral antistaphylococcal agent might be of help.
         1. Dicloxacillin (Dynapen) 500 mg PO QID
      ii. May need incision and drainage, especially if infection is progressive; culture specimen.

2.56

URINARY INCONTINENCE

I. Evaluation
   a. General—involuntary loss of urine that is often underdiagnosed and underreported.

b. Epidemiology—♀ > ♂; old > young; >25 million Americans suffer from urinary incontinence.
c. Risk factors—age, postchildbirth, and postpelvic surgery
d. Diagnostic algorithm
  i. Obtain a 24-hour bladder diary that includes fluid intake, urinary episodes, and accidents.
  ii. Determine postvoid residual (PVR) volume; if >100 mL, then abnormal.
  iii. Perform a complete abdominal and pelvic examination; assess lumbosacral nerve roots.
  iv. Obtain a urinalysis and urine culture.
    1. Treat for urinary tract infection (UTI) if applicable.
    2. Screen for diabetes if glucose is found on the urinalysis; treat if applicable.
e. Classification

NOTE:

Approximately 80% of urinary incontinence is due to stress and/or urge incontinence.

---

  i. Stress incontinence
    1. Clinical—involuntary loss of urine during an increase in intraabdominal pressure
      a. Activities include coughing, laughing, sneezing, lifting, exercise, and so on.
    2. Mechanism—weakness of the urethral sphincter muscle from
      a. Failure of anatomic supports and therefore displacement of the bladder base
      b. Loss of bladder neck competence (may occur during vaginal delivery)
      c. Intrinsic weakness of the urethral sphincter muscle (age, decreased estrogen levels, etc.)
    3. Diagnostic algorithm
      a. Limit drugs that worsen stress incontinence.
        i. For example—α_1-blockers, angiotensin-converting enzyme (ACE)-inhibitors
    4. Treatment
      a. Nonpharmacologic options
        i. Pelvic muscle exercises (Kegel's)
        ii. Weighted vaginal cones
        iii. Pelvic floor electrical stimulation
        iv. Occlusive devices (e.g., Pessaries)
      b. Pharmacologic options
        i. Localized estrogens (thicken the urethral mucosa)
          1. Premarin vaginal cream .5 to 2 g PV daily

        2. Estradiol vaginal ring (Estring)—insert PV q3mo
- ii. α_1-Agonists
  1. Pseudoephedrine (Sudafed) 15 to 30 mg PO TID
- c. Surgical options
  - i. Retropubic urethropexies
    1. For example—Burch laparoscopic and Marshall-Marchetti-Krantz (MMK) procedures
  - ii. Suburethral slings (may be minimally invasive)
  - iii. Periurethral injection at the bladder neck
- ii. Urge incontinence (overactive bladder [OAB])
  1. Clinical—involuntary loss of urine occurring when one feels the urge to urinate.
     a. Bladder may or may not be full; typically unpredictable and sudden.
  2. Mechanism—two possibilities
     a. Inappropriate bladder contraction (detrusor instability)
     b. Inappropriate relaxation of pelvic floor and sphincter muscles
  3. Diagnostic algorithm
     a. Obtain a urinalysis and urine culture to rule out UTI.
     b. Limit drugs that worsen urge incontinence.
        i. For example—diuretics, caffeine, alcohol
  4. Treatment
     a. Nonpharmacologic options
        i. Behavioral therapy, including biofeedback
        ii. Pelvic floor electrical stimulation
        iii. Extracorporeal magnetic innervation (noninvasive)
     b. Pharmacologic options
        i. Antispasmodic (typically antagonize acetylcholine receptors)
           1. Oxybutynin (Ditropan) 5 mg PO BID to QID
              Oxybutynin XL (Ditropan XL) 5 to 30 mg PO daily
           2. Tolterodine (Detrol) 1 to 2 mg PO BID
              Tolterodine ER (Detrol LA) 2 to 4 mg PO daily
           3. Hyoscyamine (Cystospaz) 0.15 to 0.3 mg PO QID
           4. Propantheline (Pro-Banthine) 7.5 to 15 mg PO q6h
           5. Dicyclomine (Bentyl) 10 to 20 mg PO QID
        ii. Tricyclic antidepressants (TCAs)
           1. Imipramine (Tofranil) 10 to 75 mg PO qhs

        iii. Localized estrogens (thicken the urethral mucosa)
          1. Premarin vaginal cream .5 to 2 g PV daily
          2. Estradiol vaginal ring (Estring)—insert PV q3mo
    c. Surgical options
      i. Implantation of sacral nerve root neuromodulator

iii. Overflow incontinence ("Paradoxical incontinence")
    1. Clinical—involuntary loss of urine usually seen with bladder (detrusor) overdistention.
      a. Patients typically have frequent dribbling of urine at any time.

NOTE:

Overflow incontinence is also called *paradoxical incontinence* as it is associated with urinary retention, high post-void residual volumes, and can usually be cured by relieving an obstructed bladder outlet.

---

    2. Mechanism—pressure from the overdistended bladder exceeds urethral pressure.
    3. Etiology (of bladder overdistension)
      a. Underactive detrusor muscle
        i. Medications
          1. Psychotropics
          2. Anticholinergics (including TCAs)
          3. Narcotics
          4. α_1- and β-agonists
          5. Calcium-channel blocker (CCB)
        ii. Rule out diabetic neuropathy, B_{12} deficiency, Parkinson's disease, multiple sclerosis (MS), spinal cord injury or disc disease, spinal stenosis, tumor, and so on.
      b. Outlet obstruction
        i. ♀—may result from pelvic organ prolapse, prior surgery, medications, and so on.
        ii. ♂—may be caused by an enlarged prostate, urethral stricture, medications, and so on.
    4. Treatment
      a. Nonpharmacologic options
        i. Scheduled reminders
        ii. Intermittent or chronic catheterization for an acontractile bladder
      b. Limit medications that may worsen patient's condition.
        i. If urinary retention is secondary to anticholinergic medications

       1. Bethanechol (Urecholine) 10 to 50 mg PO TID to QID
         a. Give 5 to 10 mg PO q1h until response, up to 50 mg.
         b. Take on an empty stomach.
     c. If urinary retention is secondary to benign prostatic hypertrophy (BPH)
       i. Pharmacologic options
         1. α_1-Antagonists (relaxes smooth muscle of prostate)
           a. Terazosin (Hytrin) 1 to 20 mg PO qhs
           b. Doxazosin (Cardura) 1 to 8 mg PO qhs
           c. Tamsulosin (Flomax) 0.4 mg PO daily

           Note: Take Tamsulosin 30 minutes after any meal.

         2. 5-α reductase inhibition (halts prostatic growth)
           a. Finasteride (Proscar) 5 mg PO daily
       ii. Surgical options
         1. Transurethral microwave thermotherapy
         2. Transurethral needle ablation
         3. Transurethral resection of the prostate (TURP)
           a. "Gold standard"
   iv. Extraurethral leakage
     1. Clinical—involuntary loss of urine from an area other than the urethra.
     2. Mechanism—most commonly caused by a fistula in the developed world.
     3. Risk factors—pelvic surgery that may result in fistula formation.
     4. Treatment—consider surgical correction.
   v. Functional incontinence (diagnosis of exclusion)
     1. Clinical—impairment in physical or cognitive function results in incontinence
     2. Treatment—scheduled reminders

II. Psychiatric pearls, pointers, and parallels
   a. Urinary incontinence may be secondary to the following
     i. UTI, especially in the elderly
       1. The elderly patient with a UTI often presents with delirium.
     ii. Normal pressure hydrocephalus (NPH)
       1. NPH triad—"wet, wacky, wobbly" (urinary incontinence, dementia, wide-based ataxic gait)
     iii. Epileptic or nonepileptic seizure

URINARY TRACT INFECTION

I. Evaluation
   a. General—urinary tract infections (UTIs) include asymptomatic bacteriuria, cystitis, pyelonephritis, and urosepsis

II. Asymptomatic bacteriuria
   a. Description—>100,000 colony-forming units (CFU) per mL of bacteria in voided urine with no clinical symptoms of UTI
   b. Etiology: *Escherichia coli, Staphylococcus saprophyticus, Proteus mirabilis, Klebsiella pneumoniae*
   c. Epidemiology—those patients who benefit from treatment for asymptomatic bacteriuria include
      i. Pregnant women
      ii. Those with renal transplants
      iii. Those scheduled for a genitourinary tract procedure
   d. Treatment—treat for 3 to 7 days using one of these agents
      i. Amoxicillin (Amoxil) 250 mg PO q8h
      ii. Cephalexin (Keflex) 500 mg PO q12h
      iii. Nitrofurantoin (Macrodantin) 100 mg PO q6h
   Note: After treatment is completed, culture urine to ensure cure and thereby avoid relapse.

REMEMBER:

Tetracyclines and fluoroquinolones are to be avoided in pregnancy.

III. Cystitis
   a. Description—inflammation of the bladder
   b. Clinical—urinary frequency, burning, hematuria, and suprapubic pain
   c. Etiology—*E. coli, S. saprophyticus, P. mirabilis, K. pneumoniae*
   d. Classification
      i. Acute uncomplicated cystitis in young women
         1. Criteria—urinalysis → pyuria (+ leukocyte esterase, + nitrite); culture not needed.

NOTE:

Not all bacteria (e.g., *S. saprophyticus*, *Enterococci*, and *Acinetobacter* species) reduce nitrates to nitrite.

---

         2. Epidemiology—those at highest risk are sexually active young women.
         3. Treatment—treat for 3 days using one of these agents

    a. Trimethoprim-sulfamethoxazole (TMP-SMZ) DS (Bactrim DS)—one tablet PO BID

    b. Ciprofloxacin (Cipro) 250 mg PO q12h

    c. Amoxicillin-clavulanate (Augmentin) 500/125 mg PO q12h

    d. Nitrofurantoin (Macrodantin) 100 mg PO q6h (may need 7 days of treatment)

NOTE:

TMP-SMZ DS (Bactrim DS) is the most cost-effective treatment and the treatment of choice for uncomplicated cystitis in young women except in areas where TMP-SMZ resistance is high.

---

  ii. Recurrent cystitis in young women

    1. Criteria—recurrent UTI and a urine culture with >100 CFU per mL of bacteria

      a. Recurrence implies that the infection is from a different organism.

    2. Treatment—as for acute uncomplicated cystitis, except treat for 7 to 10 days

    3. Prevention—for those with more than three cystitis episodes per year, consider

      a. Self-treatment with 3 days of standard therapy for each acute episode

      b. Postcoital prophylaxis if UTIs are associated with intercourse

        i. TMP-SMZ SS (Bactrim SS)

      c. Daily prophylaxis (continuously for 6 months)

        i. TMP-SMZ SS (Bactrim SS)—half tablet PO daily

        ii. Nitrofurantoin (Macrodantin) 50–100 mg PO qhs

        iii. Cephalexin (Keflex) 250 mg PO daily

  iii. Acute cystitis in men

    1. Criteria—>1,000 CFU per mL of bacteria on urine culture

    2. Epidemiology—mostly seen in those with disease of the prostate or obstruction

      a. Less often seen in young men who have anal sex or are uncircumcised.

    3. Treatment—treat for 7 to 10 days using one of these agents

      a. TMP-SMZ DS (Bactrim DS)—one tablet PO BID

      b. Ciprofloxacin (Cipro) 250 mg PO q12h

    4. Complications

      a. If bacterial prostatitis is the cause, then 6 to 12 weeks of treatment are needed.

IV. Acute uncomplicated pyelonephritis

  a. Description—inflammation of the kidney

b. Clinical
    i. Local—flank pain, symptoms of cystitis (frequency, burning, hematuria, and suprapubic pain)
    ii. Systemic—fever, chills, nausea, vomiting, abdominal pain, and leukocytosis
c. Etiology: *E. coli, S. saprophyticus, P. mirabilis, K. pneumoniae*
d. Criteria—urinalysis → pyuria (+ leukocyte esterase, + nitrite) and/or white blood cells (WBC) casts; urine culture
    i. Obtain blood cultures to rule out bacteremia.
e. Treatment—treat for 14 days using one of these agents
    i. For mild-moderate symptoms in those able to tolerate PO
        1. Treat gram negative (or empiric) with ciprofloxacin (Cipro) 500 mg PO q12h.
        2. Treat gram positive with amoxicillin-clavulanate (Augmentin) 875/125 mg PO q12h.
    ii. For severe symptoms or those who are initially unable to take PO (later can switch to PO)
        1. Ceftriaxone (Rocephin) 1 g IV/IM daily
        2. Ciprofloxacin (Cipro) 400 mg IV q12h

V. Complicated urinary tract infection
    a. Description—recurrent, persistent UTIs in the setting of anatomic, functional, or medication factors
    b. Clinical—ranges from cystitis to urosepsis
    c. Etiology—*E. coli, P. mirabilis, K. pneumoniae, Enterococcus* species, *Pseudomonas aeruginosa*
    d. Criteria—>10,000 CFU per mL of bacteria on urine culture
    e. Treatment—treat for 10 to 14 days using one of these agents
        i. For mild-moderate symptoms in those able to tolerate PO
            1. Treat gram negative with ciprofloxacin (Cipro) 500 mg PO q12h.
            2. Treat *Enterococcus* species with ampicillin (Principen) 500 mg PO q6h.
        ii. For severe symptoms or those who are initially unable to take PO (cover Pseudomonas)
            1. Cefepime (Maxipime) 1 to 2 g IV/IM q12h
            2. Piperacillin-tazobactam (Zosyn) 3.375 g IV q6h
            3. Meropenem (Merrem) 1 g IV q8h
            4. Aztreonam (Azactam) 0.5 to 2 g IV/IM q8h to q12h
        iii. For Vancomycin-resistant *Enterococcus faecium*, consider linezolid (Zyvox) 600 mg IV/PO q12h
    Note: After treatment is completed, culture urine to ensure cure and thereby avoid relapse.

VI. Catheter-associated urinary tract infection
    a. Description—indwelling Foley catheters increase the risk of bacteriuria by 5% per day
    b. Etiology—varied, and typically polymicrobial
    c. Criteria—>100 CFU per mL of bacteria on urine culture
    d. Treatment—remove the catheter; treat *symptomatic* bacteriuria for 10 to 14 days using

      i. If gram negative, treat with ciprofloxacin (Cipro) 500 mg PO q12h.

      ii. If gram positive, treat with ampicillin (Principen) 500 mg PO q6h.

> **NOTE:**
>
> In general, treatment is not necessary for catheterized patients who have asymptomatic bacteriuria; exceptions include the immunosuppressed, those at risk for endocarditis, and those scheduled for a genitourinary procedure.

VII. Urinary tract pain
    a. Analgesia for dysuria (pain or burning on urination)
      i. Phenazopyridine (Pyridium) 100 to 200 mg PO TID (after meals) × 2 days
        1. Turns urine red/orange
VIII. Psychiatric pearls, pointers, and parallels
    a. Include a urinalysis as part of the delirium work-up to rule out a UTI.
      i. Recall that elderly patients with a UTI often present with delirium.

2.58

VAGINITIS

I. Evaluation
    a. General—inflammation of the vagina
    b. Etiology
      i. Bacterial vaginosis (40%–50% of cases)
        1. Clinical—adherent and malodorous ("fishy") off-white discharge
          a. *NO* dyspareunia, pruritus, or inflammation; many ♀ are asymptomatic.
        2. Etiology—change in vaginal flora
          a. Decrease in normal vaginal bacteria (lactobacillus)
          b. Increase in Gardnerella vaginalis, and so on.
        3. Epidemiology—most common type of vaginitis in child-bearing women
        4. Risk factors—nonwhite, previous pregnancy, intrauterine device (IUD)
        5. Diagnosis—increase in vaginal pH (>4.5), clue cells (epithelial cells covered with bacteria)

      a. No need for culture.
6. Treatment
    a. Metronidazole (Flagyl) 500 mg PO BID × 7 days
    b. Metronidazole (Flagyl) 2 g PO × one dose (higher recurrence rates vs. 7-day treatment)
    c. Metronidazole (Metrogel) vaginal .75% gel—PV qhs OR BID × 5 days
    d. Clindamycin (ClindaMax) vaginal 2% cream—PV qhs × 3 to 7 days
7. Recurrent bacterial vaginosis
    a. General—approximately 30% who previously responded have recurrence in 3 months
    b. Treatment—10 to 14 days of therapy is required for symptomatic relapse.
8. Complications
    a. Increased risk of premature birth (15%–20% pregnant women affected).
    b. Consider checking human immunodeficiency virus (HIV) status in these patients.
ii. Candidal vulvovaginitis (20%–25% of cases)
    1. Clinical—pruritus, vaginal discomfort, curd-like discharge, and painful coitus
        a. White plaques on vaginal walls, vulvar erythema, and edema

---

NOTE:

As many as 50% of women given the diagnosis of candidal vulvovaginitis may have other diagnoses; therefore, it is best to make the specific diagnosis of vaginitis utilizing microscopy and vaginal culture, if needed.

---

    2. Etiology—*Candida albicans* (80%–92%), *Candida glabrata*
    3. Epidemiology—common in women of childbearing age
    4. Risk factors—diabetes, antibiotics, steroids, HIV, ↑ estrogen levels (oral contraceptive pills [OCPs], pregnancy)
        a. Also, vaginal sponge and IUD
    5. Diagnosis—normal vaginal pH (4.0–4.5), pseudohyphae on 10% potassium hydroxide (KOH)
    6. Treatment
        a. Topical antimycotic agents (cure rate = ~80%)
            i. Clotrimazole vaginal creams
                1. One percent = Mycelex-7/Gyne-Lotrimin 7—PV qhs × 7 days
                2. Two percent = Gyne-Lotrimin 3—PV qhs × 3 days
            ii. Miconazole vaginal creams (or suppository)
                1. Two percent = Monistat 7 (or 100 mg suppository)—PV qhs × 7 days

   2. Four percent = monistat 3 (or 200 mg suppos-
      itory)—PV qhs × 3 days
b. Oral antimycotic agents
   i. Fluconazole (Diflucan) 150 mg PO × one dose
   Note: Oral azoles such as fluconazole are contraindicated
   in pregnancy.

7. Complicated candidal vulvovaginitis (typically in those
   with risk factors listed in the preceding text)
   a. Risk factors—diabetes, antibiotic therapy, recurrent
      candidiasis, *C. glabrata* infection.
   b. Treatment—10 to 14 days of therapy

8. Recurrent candidal vulvovaginitis
   a. General—more than four episodes of infection in
      1 year
   b. Etiology—unclear; biologic susceptibility versus sex-
      ual transmission versus decreased immunity
   c. Treatment
      i. Oral antimycotic maintenance suppressive ther-
         apy (for 6 months)
         1. Fluconazole (Diflucan) 100 mg PO weekly
         2. Itraconazole (Sporanox) 50 to 100 mg PO
            daily
   d. Complications—consider checking HIV status in
      these patients

iii. Trichomoniasis (15%–20% of cases)
    1. Clinical—purulent and malodorous discharge, painful
       coitus, and vulvovaginal erythema
    2. Etiology—trichomonas vaginalis
    3. Epidemiology—Affects 2 to 3 million American women
       per year
    4. Diagnosis—increase in vaginal pH (5.0–6.0), neutrophils
       and motile trichomonads on microscopy
    5. Treatment—(cure rate = ~85% with either)
       a. Metronidazole (Flagyl) 500 mg PO BID × 7 days
       b. Metronidazole (Flagyl) 2 g PO × one dose
       Note: Do not use metronidazole in the first trimester
       of pregnancy. Additionally, beware that metronidazole
       interacts with alcohol (disulfiram-reaction) and warfarin.

REMEMBER:

Treat sexual partners simultaneously as the cure rate then increases to
>90%.

---

    6. Recurrent/refractory trichomoniasis
       a. Treatment—metronidazole (Flagyl) 500 mg to 1 g
          PO q6h × 10 to 14 days

7. Complications—assists in HIV transmission; therefore, consider checking HIV status.

iv. Gonococcal vaginitis/cervicitis
1. Clinical—urethritis initially → cervicitis, yellowish/bloody discharge, and dysuria
   a. Asymptomatic in 50% to 80% of affected women.

REMEMBER:

Ten to fifteen percent of infected women will develop pelvic inflammatory disease (PID), which can result in infertility; therefore, treat early, and treat sexual partners to avoid reinfection.

---

2. Etiology—*Neisseria gonorrhoeae*
3. Epidemiology—>300,000 cases of gonorrhea reported annually in the United States
   a. Gonorrhea is the no. 2 reported communicable infection (Chlamydia is no. 1).

NOTE:

From a single act of intercourse, a woman has approximately 50% chance of acquiring gonorrhea from an infected man; in the converse scenario, a man is approximately 20% likely to acquire gonorrhea from an infected woman.

---

4. Diagnosis—culture required as false-negative rate for cervical smears is 60% to 70%
5. Treatment
   a. Ceftriaxone (Rocephin) 125 mg IM × one dose
   b. Ciprofloxacin (Cipro) 500 mg PO × one dose
   c. Doxycycline (Vibramycin) 100 mg PO BID × 7 days
      i. Chlamydia infection often coexists, which doxycycline treats
6. Complications—test for chlamydia in all patients; offer HIV testing

v. Atrophic vaginitis
1. Clinical—vaginal dryness, erythema, and thinning; painful coitus; and postcoital burn are the findings.
2. Etiology—epithelium thins from decreased endogenous estrogen; vaginal milieu changes.
3. Epidemiology—clinically significant disease is rare.
4. Diagnosis—increase in vaginal pH (>6.0), mixed flora and gram-negative rods on smear.
5. Treatment—topical vaginal estrogen; recurrence may require systemic estrogen.

II. Psychiatric pearls, pointers, and parallels
a. Trauma/abuse

    i. Vaginitis may be a "simple" infection, but may also be a clue to physical or sexual trauma.

        1. Inquire about trauma/abuse in a nonthreatening manner.

        2. Send patient for a rape kit (further testing for sexually transmitted diseases) if necessary.

2.59

WOUND CARE

I. Cleaning the wound

  a. General

    i. Clean wounds as soon as possible to prevent bacterial counts from reaching infective levels.

  b. Preparation

    i. All wound care should be done with the patient supine because fainting commonly occurs.

    ii. Utilize universal precautions including protective eyewear and a mask.

    iii. Attend to patient comfort with appropriate local/systemic anesthetic.

  c. Methods of wound cleaning

    i. Mechanical scrubbing

        1. First, scrub a wide area of skin around the wound with antiseptic.

        2. Scrubbing the wound itself could be abrasive and lead to more tissue damage.

          a. Therefore, one may choose to irrigate first and scrub if contaminants remain.

    ii. Irrigation

        1. Delivering irrigation fluid at a higher pressure is most effective for cleaning.

        2. Some emergency medicine studies show tap water had less of an infection rate than sterile saline.

        3. Antibiotic solutions have been used for irrigation.

  d. Agents of wound cleaning

    i. Skin antiseptics—use only to clean intact skin; avoid significant amounts in open wounds

        1. Povidone-iodine solution (Betadine 10%)

          a. General—virucidal and bactericidal

b. Uses—at 10%, use in periphery; dilute to 1% for wound irrigation

2. Chlorhexidine gluconate (Hibiclens)
   a. General—bactericidal (better against gram-positive than gram-negative bacteria)
   b. Uses—hand cleanser; avoid use for wounds that are open

3. Hydrogen peroxide (H_2O_2)
   a. General—weak antibacterial
   b. Uses—superficial lacerations/abrasions; toxic to tissue and hemolytic

ii. Antibiotic solutions

e. Wound closure
   i. For superficial lacerations/abrasions, may apply bacitracin and dressing or leave open.
      1. For abrasions, consider applying zinc oxide BID to promote healing.
   ii. For lacerations, may need surgical consult.
      1. Simple deep lacerations may only need cleaning, sutures, or steri-strips.
         a. For these, use antibiotic ointment and dressing BID × 7 to 10 days.
      2. More complex lacerations require exploration of the wound's full extent.
         a. Rule out hidden foreign bodies, structural injuries, and so on.
         b. Employ debridement and/or excision if significant contamination exists.
            i. Do NOT suture infected wounds → a closed-space infection may develop.
            ii. Therefore, make sure wounds are fully explored, cleaned, and so on before closure.

f. Tetanus toxoid
   i. Adult formulations (for those 7 years or older)
      1. Td (tetanus and diphtheria toxoids adsorbed) 0.5 mL IM
   ii. Primary immunization and booster
      1. Primary—Td × two doses 4 to 8 weeks apart, and then one dose 6 to 12 months later
      2. Booster—Td q10yr
   Note: A fourth dose of tetanus toxoid completes the initial series
   iii. Prophylaxis and treatment in wound care
      1. For clean, minor wounds
         a. Give Td if >10 years since last dose (assuming prior immunization).
         b. Give Td if patient never got a fourth dose of tetanus toxoid.

2. For contaminated wounds, puncture wounds, burns, and so on
    a. Give Td if >5 years since last dose (assuming prior immunization).
    b. Give Td and immune globulin if patient never got a fourth dose of toxoid.

II. Bite wounds
  a. General—can result from any animal source, including humans.
  b. Clinical—laceration injury, signs of infection appear within 3 days from direct inoculation of microorganisms.
  c. Etiology—wounds contain polymicrobial flora.

> **NOTE:**
>
> Bite wounds contain the aerobic and anaerobic flora from the biter's oral cavity and the victim's skin.

  i. Common microbes isolated
    1. Human
        a. Gram-positive bacteria (*Staphylococcus aureus, viridans streptococci, peptostreptococci*)
        b. Gram-negative rods (*Prevotella, Bacteroides, Fusobacterium, Eikenella*)
    2. Dog and cat
        a. Gram-positive bacteria (*S. aureus, Staphylococcus intermedius*)
        b. Gram-negative rods
            i. *Pasteurella multocida* and other *pasteurella* species
            ii. *Haemophilus felix*
            iii. *Capnocytophaga*
            iv. *Porphyromonas*
            v. Prevotella
            vi. *Bacteroides*
        c. Gram-negative cocci (*Neisseria canis*)
  d. Epidemiology—>1,000,000 of those suffering animal bites present for medical treatment
  e. Treatment
    i. Wound management as described in the preceding text (including tetanus toxoid as outlined in the preceding text)
    ii. Pharmacologic treatment
        1. Medication options

> **NOTE:**
>
> Use of penicillin for bite infections may be inadequate because >40% of bite wounds contain β-lactamase-producing microorganisms.

        a. Amoxicillin-clavulanate (Augmentin) 500/125 mg PO q8h

      b. Doxycycline (Vibramycin) 100 mg PO BID

      c. Moxifloxacin (Avelox) 400 mg PO daily + Clindamycin (Cleocin) 300 to 600 mg PO q6h

      d. Ceftriaxone (Rocephin) 1 to 2 g IM/IV daily (for compliance concerns)

  2. Duration

    a. Prophylactic = 3 to 7 days

    b. Soft tissue/frank cellulitis = 10 to 14 days

    c. Joints or bone involvement = 21 days minimum

  iii. Additional cautions

    1. For human bites, determine medical status of the biter (human immunodeficiency virus [HIV], hepatitis, rapid plasma reagin [RPR]).

      a. Test the victim at the time of the incident and 6 months later

      b. Prophylactic treatment of the victim as indicated

    2. For dog and other animal bites, rule out rabies.

      a. Victims of a nonprovoked animal are at higher risk for rabies.

      b. Determine animal's vaccination status against rabies.

      c. Observe/quarantine the animal in question for 10 days.

      d. If rabies is suspected, or animal cannot be located, then treat the victim.

        i. Begin rabies series within 48 hours of the bite.

          1. Rabies immune globulin 20 IU per kg

          2. Rabies vaccine on days 0, 3, 7, 14, and 28

        ii. If victim had rabies vaccination previously, then

          1. No need for rabies immune globulin.

          2. Rabies vaccine on days 0 and 3

Note: This sequence can stop if animal is proved to be rabies free.

III. Decubitus ulcers (pressure ulcers/bed sores)

  a. General—lesion that results from continual pressure causing damage to underlying tissue.

  b. Clinical—usually occurs in soft tissue overlying a bony area.

    i. Classification as proposed by the National Pressure Ulcer Advisory Panel (see Table 2.59.1)

  c. Etiology

    i. Pressure—perpendicular force adversely affecting tissue (typically at a bony area)

    ii. Shear—parallel force adversely affecting tissue (e.g., patient slides in bed)

    iii. Friction—adherent force that resists shear

  d. Epidemiology—1.6 million such ulcers developed in US hospitals (Beckrich & Aronovich, 1999)

  e. Risk factors—moisture, irritants, old age, limited movement, poor nutrition, steroids, smoking, diabetes, and so on

  f. Differential diagnosis

TABLE 2.59.1 National Pressure Ulcer Advisory Panel Classification of Decubitus Ulcers

Stage	Description
I	Pressure-related change of unbroken skin
II	Partial-thickness skin loss affecting the epidermis ± dermis
III	Full-thickness skin loss involving subcutaneous tissue extending as far as fascia
IV	Full-thickness skin loss with damage to muscle, bone, or other structures

In order to stage an ulcer, one must see the bottom of the wound; otherwise, the stage of the ulcer cannot be classified.
Adapted from Niezgoda JA, Mendez-Eastman S. The effective management of pressure ulcers. *Adv Skin Wound Care.* 2006;19(Suppl 1):3–15.

    i. Arterial ulcers—found on distal digits or over a bony area.

    ii. Diabetic ulcers—found on calloused areas.

    iii. Venous stasis ulcers—found on the lateral region of the lower extremities.

g. Management

    i. Relieve pressure.

       1. Change the patient's body position often; turning and positioning are key factors.

       2. Reduce tissue-to-surface contact with either static or dynamic devices.

          a. Pillows or boot devices may decrease heel pressure.

          b. For multiple bed sores, consider a low-air-loss bed or air-fluidized bed.

    ii. Assess and relieve pain.

    iii. Assess and provide adequate nutrition and hydration.

       1. Adjust calories to account for stress; therefore, 30 to 35 kcal/kg/day.

       2. Higher healing rates occur with increased protein intake of 1.2 to 1.5 g/kg/day.

       3. Assure for adequate intake of vitamins and minerals; supplement if needed.

       4. Adequate hydration requires 30 mL/kg/day of water.

    iv. Remove necrotic debris utilizing any of the following options:

       1. Surgical debridement—typically utilized for infected ulcers.

       2. Mechanical debridement—moist gauze adheres by drying; removal then debrides.

       3. Enzymatic (chemical) debridement—digests devitalized tissue.

          a. For example, collagenase, papain/urea with or without chlorophyll

4. Autolytic debridement—uses body's own endogenous enzymes at wound surface.
5. Biologic debridement—uses medical maggots to feed on devitalized tissue.

v. Maintain a moist wound setting.
1. Change gauze frequently to prevent drying.
2. Polymer film or hydrocolloid dressings can be used for stage I and II ulcers.
   a. For example, DuoDerm (hydrocolloid)—apply q5d.
      i. Interacts with wound exudate—gel; therefore, removes easily
3. Alginates or hydrogel dressings can be used for stage III and IV ulcers.

vi. Promote formation of granulation tissue; allow for re-epithelialization to occur.
1. Limit antiseptic agents to infected ulcers because they are also toxic to native tissue.

vii. Control infection
1. Bacterial colonization at an ulcer site does not equate to infection.
2. Diagnose infection based on erythema, edema, pain, warmth, fever, exudate, and so on.
   a. Treat with oral or IV antibiotics depending on severity.

h. Prevention
i. Keep patients clean and dry.
ii. For those patients who are immobile, turn them every hour.
iii. Examine at pressure points (e.g., heel, sacrum) for signs of ulcer formation.

Part 3

Some Important Psychiatric Syndromes

SYNDROME OF INAPPROPRIATE SECRETION OF ANTIDIURETIC HORMONE

I. Antidiuretic hormone (ADH) overview
   a. ADH, also called *vasopressin*, is a hormone synthesized in the hypothalamus.
   b. It is stored in the pituitary gland.
   c. Release is regulated by central nervous system (CNS) and chest baroreceptors, which detect changes in blood volume and pressure.
   d. ADH acts on the kidneys to increase total body water.
   e. Secretion normally occurs in the presence of hypovolemia.
   f. ADH secretion in euvolemic patients results in syndrome of inappropriate secretion of antidiuretic hormone (SIADH), with increased excretion of sodium, resulting in hyponatremia, and retention of water.

II. Causes
   a. Pulmonary diseases, especially pneumonia
   b. CNS illnesses—stroke, hemorrhage, traumatic injury, infection
   c. Paraneoplastic production of ADH by a tumor
   d. Certain chemotherapy agents
   e. Exogenous administration of vasopressin or desmopressin
   f. Psychiatric medications
      i. Antipsychotic medications
      ii. Antidepressant medications such as tricyclics, monoamine oxidase inhibitors, and selective serotonin reuptake inhibitors
      iii. Anticonvulsants and mood stabilizers—carbamazepine and oxcarbazepine

III. Clinical features
   a. Symptoms generally occur only when hyponatremia is severe, that is, ≤ 120 to 125 mEq per L.
   b. Early symptoms include malaise, anorexia; gastrointestinal symptoms such as nausea, vomiting, diarrhea; muscle cramps.
   c. Late symptoms are due to CNS effects of hyponatremia—headache, blurred vision, irritability, lethargy, confusion, deteriorating mental status, decreased reflexes, seizure, coma.
   d. Death may also occur.

IV. Laboratory findings
   a. Low plasma sodium, that is, hyponatremia
   b. High urine sodium (>40 mEq/L)

c. Low plasma osmolality (<280 mOsm/kg)
d. High urine osmolality (>150 to 200 mOsm/kg)
e. Low to normal blood urea nitrogen (BUN)
f. Hypouricemia (<4 mg/dL)
g. Normal potassium
h. High urine osmolality with a low plasma osmolality in the absence of diuretic use is confirmatory.
i. Osmolality is a more precise measurement of urine concentration than specific gravity, although the specific gravity will also be similarly affected.

V. Treatment

a. Water is restricted to 0.5 to 1 L per day (i.e., ~50% of daily requirement) in asymptomatic hyponatremia or chronic SIADH.
b. Salt administration with hypertonic saline (3% sodium chloride intravenous) if symptomatic. Add a loop diuretic (furosemide) because the sodium chloride alone will be excreted in the urine but the water will be retained in SIADH, and can worsen the hyponatremia. The diuretic will help get rid of some of the water and create a negative free-water balance.
c. In refractory cases, demeclocycline 300 to 600 mg PO BID can be used to induce a negative free-water balance.
d. Medication-induced SIADH will generally respond to stopping the drug, and restriction of fluids.

REMEMBER:

Do not correct the hyponatremia too rapidly because doing so can lead to central pontine myelinolysis. The initial aim of treatment is to bring the sodium level to 125 to 130 mEq per L. If the patient is asymptomatic, raise plasma sodium at 0.5 mEq per L per hour. If symptomatic, raise it at 1.0 to 1.5 mEq/L/hour for the first few hours, then slow down the rate of administration.

VI. Psychogenic polydipsia with secondary hyponatremia

NOTE:

In the psychiatric patient, psychogenic polydipsia with secondary hyponatremia will give rise to a picture similar to SIADH.

---

a. Psychogenic polydipsia with secondary hyponatremia may coexist with SIADH.
b. Patients with primary polydipsia have normal suppression of ADH and have dilute urine.
c. If the urine osmolality is high, then there is likely pathologic ADH release or sensitivity.
d. Strict measurement of daily water intake, and 24 hours urine collection may point to polydipsia.

    i.   Abnormal diurnal weight gain of 1.2% over the morning weight is a sign of water intoxication. Use the following formula to obtain the diurnal weight gain percentage:

(4:00 PM weight–7:00 AM weight) divided by 7:00 AM weight, multiplied by 100.

    ii.   Weight gains of 7% or more is associated with plasma sodium concentrations of <125 mmol per L

3.2

NEUROLEPTIC MALIGNANT SYNDROME

I. Neuroleptic malignant syndrome (NMS) overview
   a. Life-threatening condition caused by antipsychotic medications, including the new generation antipsychotic medications.
   b. Reported in patients on tricyclic antidepressants.
   c. Also seen in patients who are rapidly withdrawn from dopamine agonists such as antiparkinsonian medications.
   d. Generally occurs during the first week to a month on the treatment, although it can develop at any time during treatment.
   e. Typically takes 1 to 3 days to develop fully.
   f. May last from a few hours to a few weeks.
   g. It can be fatal.
   h. Risk factors
      i. High-potency antipsychotic
      ii. High-dose antipsychotic
      iii. Prior NMS
      iv. Rapid dose increase
      v. Age younger than 40 years
      vi. Males
      vii. Dehydration, malnutrition
II. Criteria for the diagnosis of NMS
   a. Hyperthermia—oral temperature of at least $38°$ C in the absence of other causes of fever
   b. Muscle rigidity, which is generally of the lead pipe type, although it can also be of the cogwheel variety.
   c. Several of the following:
      i. Altered mental status—altered sensorium, confusion, disorientation, stupor, coma

    ii. Autonomic instability—increased pulse, increased respiration, increased systolic and/or diastolic blood pressure, diaphoresis, urinary incontinence

    iii. Extrapyramidal symptoms—resting tremor, oculogyric crisis, choreiform movements, flexor-extensor posturing, festinating gait, sialorrhea, dysphagia

    iv. Laboratory abnormal findings:

NOTE:

Laboratory findings are similar to those seen in dehydration states, renal failure, and rhabdomyolysis, which are potential complications of NMS.

---

        1. Elevated creatinine kinase levels ($>1,000$ IU/mL) due to extreme muscle rigidity and contractility

        2. Leukocytosis ($>15,000$ white cells/mm^3)

        3. Metabolic acidosis

        4. Increased transaminases

III. Treatment

  a. Stop the offending agent immediately.

  b. Use supportive measures (hydration, cooling, oxygen).

  c. Moderate to severe NMS should be referred to an acute medical treatment facility.

  d. Rule out other causes for fever.

  e. The following medications have been useful according to some studies, but unsafe according to others:

    i. Amantadine (Symmetrel) 100 mg PO BID. Dose may be increased to 200 mg PO BID.

    ii. Dopamine agonist bromocriptine (Parlodel) 2.5 mg to 5 mg q4h is effective for muscle rigidity and also reduces fever.

    iii. Dantroline (Dantrium) 25 to 50 mg PO BID to QID, also helps with muscle rigidity.

    iv. Some studies have found that patients who received the above medications took longer to recover and had worse sequelae than those treated by supportive means.

    v. Current data suggest that supportive measures be tried first, unless the patient's condition is moderate to severe.

  f. If refractory, may try IV benzodiazepines such as lorazepam or diazepam.

  g. An uncontrolled psychosis in the presence of NMS can be effectively treated with electroconvulsive therapy (ECT); however, safety is a concern because ECT in patients with NMS may lead to cardiac arrhythmias and cardiac arrest.

IV. Prognosis

  a. Mortality is 10% to 20%.

  b. If patient is rechallenged with an antipsychotic medication within 2 weeks of an episode, 60% will have a recurrence.

   c. If more than 2 weeks have elapsed, 30% will have a recurrence.

   d. 90% will be able to tolerate an antipsychotic at some point in the future.

   e. Use an alternate antipsychotic medication if necessary, slower titration of antipsychotic, and use proper caution, with proper monitoring for recurrence of NMS.

   f. Continue to observe the patient for recurrence of symptoms for a month after an index episode.

3.3

SEROTONIN SYNDROME

I. Overview
   a. A potentially fatal condition that results from the combination of two or more drugs that overactivate the serotonin system in the central nervous system (CNS)
   b. Characterized by mental status, autonomic, and neuromuscular changes
   c. Occurs when multiple serotonergic agents are used together, or are used in close succession
   d. Risk factors
      i. Elderly
      ii. Slow metabolizers of selective serotonin reuptake inhibitors (SSRIs)
      iii. Peripheral vascular disease

II. Medications that can cause serotonin syndrome
   a. SSRIs used together with lithium, tryptophan, dextromethorphan, trazodone
   b. Combination of monoamine oxidase inhibitors (MAOIs), SSRIs, clomipramine, or tricyclic antidepressants
   c. Clomipramine

NOTE:

Drugs such as cocaine and amphetamines can also induce serotonin syndrome by inhibiting serotonin uptake.

III. Diagnosis
   a. Onset of symptoms is within minutes to hours following an increase in dose or an addition of a serotonergic agent.

b. Change in mental status includes agitation, euphoria, drowsiness, delirium, confusion, hypomania, dizziness, psychosis, seizures, and coma.

c. Autonomic instability includes fever, diaphoresis, shivering, tachycardia, hypertension, hypotension, tachypnea, nausea, and diarrhea.

d. Neuromuscular abnormalities are hyperreflexia, clonus, tremor, increased tone, nystagmus. (Be aware that muscle rigidity can make it difficult to ascertain hyperreflexia and clonus.)

e. Rule out other causes of fever such as infections, substance abuse or withdrawal, and metabolic disorders.

f. Consider recent use of an antipsychotic agent, to rule out neuroleptic malignant syndrome (NMS) (see Table 3.3.1).

TABLE 3.3.1 Comparison of Neuroleptic Malignant Syndrome (NMS) and Serotonin Syndrome

Factors	NMS	Serotonin Syndrome
Mechanism	Dopamine blockade	Serotonin excess
Onset	Days to weeks	Minutes to hours
Resolution	1–2 wk	<24 hr
Rhabdomyolysis	Common	unusual
Abnormal liver function tests	Common	unusual
Metabolic acidosis	Common	unusual
Leukocytosis	Common	unusual

IV. Treatment

a. Discontinue the serotonergic agent(s).

b. General supportive therapy is with hydration, external cooling, acetaminophen to control fever.

c. Severe hyperthermia, with fever of $>40.5°C$, will require more aggressive treatment.

    i. Administer antiserotonergic agent cyproheptadine 4 mg PO or through gastric tube q1h × three to four doses.

    ii. Muscular rigidity that accompanies fever may respond to benzodiazepine therapy.

    iii. Benzodiazepines (lorazepam or diazepam) are used for myoclonus, and hyperreflexia. (Clonazepam, which is not a potent $GABA_B$ receptor agonist, has not been found to be effective in the serotonin syndrome.)

    iv. Anesthesia or nondepolarizing neuromuscular blocking agents may be necessary if benzodiazepines fail to control muscle activity or seizures.

> **KEY POINT:**
>
> Dantrolene, bromocriptine, and propranolol should not be used. Dantrolene and bromocriptine may precipitate or worsen serotonin syndrome. Propranolol can cause hypotension and shock in an autonomically unstable patient.

V. Prognosis
   a. Mortality is 11%.
   b. Most cases resolve completely within 24 hours if treated appropriately.
   c. There is no need for further monitoring after an episode has resolved.
   d. Upon rechallenge, patients are at a higher risk for recurrence.
   e. Consider discontinuing combination drug treatment, using a lower dose or a lower-potency serotonergic medication.

3.4

NORADRENERGIC SYNDROME (EARLY TRICYCLIC SYNDROME)

I. Overview
   a. It occurs most often in patients with panic disorder.
   b. It involves treatment with noradrenergic medications such as desipramine and imipramine.
II. Symptoms
   a. Nervousness, restlessness, tremulousness, fever, agitation, difficulty in concentrating, insomnia, increased anxiety.
   b. Symptoms occur when the medications are started.
   c. Symptoms are usually transient.
   d. By the time the medication is therapeutic (several weeks after the medication is started), the symptoms will have resolved.
   e. Symptoms may be so uncomfortable that the patient might discontinue the medication very early in treatment.
III. Prevention
   a. Start patients with panic disorder on low doses (10–20 mg of imipramine or desipramine a day).
   b. Gradually increase dose to 150 mg per day.

c. May be prevented by adding either of the following:
  i. Propranolol 20 to 40 mg PO TID
  ii. Diazepam 5 mg PO BID or TID

REMEMBER:

Panic disorder is better treated with selective serotonin reuptake inhibitors (SSRIs).

3.5

SELECTIVE SEROTONIN REUPTAKE INHIBITORS WITHDRAWAL SYNDROME

I. Overview
  a. Symptoms begin 1to 3 days after abrupt cessation of selective serotonin reuptake inhibitors (SSRIs).
  b. It also occurs with discontinuation of the serotonin-norepinephrine reuptake inhibitor (SNRI) venlafaxine, and the serotonergic tricyclic antidepressant (clomipramine).
  c. Cause—when SSRI is discontinued, level of serotonin decreases, and is no longer able to provide a stimulus for receptors formerly downregulated while SSRI was in the system.
  d. Frequency—occurs in 25% to 30% patients who discontinue SSRI.
  e. Risks
    i. Duration of treatment >4 weeks
    ii. Higher doses of medication
    iii. SSRIs with short half-life and no active metabolite—paroxetine, fluvoxamine
    iv. Clomipramine
    v. Note that symptoms may occur weeks later if patient abruptly discontinues an SSRI with a longer half-life.
II. Diagnosis
  a. Two or more symptoms
    i. Constitutional—flu-like symptoms, malaise, chills, myalgias
    ii. Gastrointestinal—nausea, vomiting, diarrhea
    iii. Mental status changes and affecting symptoms—anxiety, irritability, mood lability, insomnia, bizarre dreams, confusion, and lethargy

   iv. Neuromuscular—dizziness, lightheadedness, vertigo, headache, tremor, dystonia, electrical shock sensation upon neck flexion (identical to Lhermitte's sign), and gait instability
   b. Symptoms develop within 1 to 7 days of discontinuation or abrupt decrease.
   c. Symptoms cause distress or impairment in functioning.
   d. Symptoms are not due to another medical condition or another substance.
   e. Symptoms are not due to recurrence or exacerbation of the primary psychiatric diagnosis.
   f. Patient must have been taking the SSRI for at least 1 month.

III. Treatment
   a. If symptoms are acute, restart the SSRI at the same dose at which medication was discontinued.
   b. Slow taper over weeks. The following is a tapering schedule commonly used:
      i. Paroxetine—reduce by 10 mg every 2 weeks until dose is 10 mg per day, then by 5 mg per day every 2 weeks.
      ii. Fluvoxamine—reduce by 25 mg every 2 weeks until dose is 25 mg per day, then by 12.5 mg every 2 weeks.
      iii. Sertraline—reduce by 25 mg every 2 weeks until dose is 25 mg per day, then by 12.5 mg every 2 weeks.
      iv. Venlafaxine—reduce by 25 mg every 2 weeks until dose is 25 mg per day, then by 12.5 mg every 2 weeks.
         1. For the extended release formulation—reduce by 37.5 mg every 2 weeks
      v. Fluoxetine—reduce by 5 mg every 2 weeks until dose is 5 mg per day, then by 2.5 mg every 2 weeks.
   c. If symptoms continue with slow taper, try cross-tapering with a medication that has a longer half-life.

REMEMBER:

If you decide to switch your patient to a monoamine oxidase inhibitor (MAOI), wait at least a week after discontinuation of the SSRI before starting the MAOI. Wait 2 weeks if the patient has been taking paroxetine or sertraline, and 5 weeks if taking fluoxetine.

IV. Prognosis
   a. Condition can resolve on its own and is not generally life-threatening.
   b. Good prognosis with treatment as described in the preceding text.

HEATSTROKE

I. Cause
   a. Occurs from a breakdown in heat regulatory mechanisms causing cessation in sweating.
   b. Major factor is increased ambient temperature, particularly with high humidity.
   c. When the body's temperature regulation fails, the core temperature keeps rising.
   d. The hyperthermia can cause multiple organ system failure.
   e. Two types
      i. Classic heatstroke—arises when the person has not exerted himself or herself.
      ii. Exertional heatstroke—arises when working or exercising in a hot environment.
         1. Medical risk factors need not be present.
         2. This type of heatstroke can occur in a healthy individual.

REMEMBER:

Heatstroke is a medical emergency. Patients may die within a few hours of onset, or in a few weeks from organ damage.

II. Risk factors
   a. Elderly
   b. Infants and children
   c. Medical conditions
      i. Congestive heart failure
      ii. Arteriosclerosis
      iii. Diabetes mellitus
      iv. Hyperthyroidism
      v. Substances—alcohol, caffeine, cocaine, heroin, and Phencyclidine (PCP)
      vi. Dermatologic/rheumatologic conditions that make it difficult to lose sweat
         1. Congenital absence of sweat glands
         2. Ectodermal dysplasia
         3. Severe scleroderma
   d. Medications
      i. Drugs that decrease heat loss
         1. Anticholinergics, phenothiazines, and antihistamines decrease sweating.
         2. Diuretics, calcium-channel blockers, and β-blockers all decrease cardiovascular reserve.

        3. Barbiturates depress the central nervous system (CNS) response to heat production.

    ii. Drugs that may increase heat production—amphetamines, neuroleptics

    iii. Drugs that depress thirst—butyrophenones

    iv. Heatstroke from lithium in combination with the selective serotonin reuptake inhibitor (SSRI) fluoxetine has been reported

III. Signs and symptoms

    a. Prodromal symptoms

      i. Generally absent

      ii. Some patients may complain of headache, vertigo, lightheadedness, abdominal distress, or confusion

    b. Skin—dry, hot

    c. Vital signs

      i. Core body temperature of at least 40.5°C (104.9°F)

        1. Core body temperature should be obtained with a rectal, esophageal, or bladder probe.

        2. Oral, tympanic, and axillary temperatures do not give an accurate core temperature reading.

        3. Rectal temperature exceeds 40.5°C (104.9°F) and may reach 44°C (112°F).

        4. Core temperature over 41°C (107°F) is often fatal.

      ii. Tachycardia of up to 160 to 180 beats per minute

      iii. Tachypnea, with weak and shallow respirations

      iv. Hypotension

    d. Neurologic/psychiatric signs

      i. Acute mental status changes—confusion, irritability, and bizarre behavior

      ii. Ataxia

      iii. Coma

      iv. Decorticate (flexor) posturing

      v. Seizures

IV. Laboratory findings

    a. Complete blood counts (CBC) is consistent with dehydration—leukocytosis, elevated hematocrit.

    b. Cardiac enzymes may be elevated due to cardiac ischemia/infarction.

    c. Fibrinogin, fibrin split products signal disseminated intravascular coagulopathy (DIC).

      i. Signs of DIC include ecchymosis, epistaxis, hematemesis, and hematuria.

    d. Abnormal liver function tests signal hepatic failure.

    e. Elevated blood urea nitrogen (BUN) and creatinine signal acute renal failure.

    f. Urinalysis, showing hematuria and myoglobin casts, are consistent with renal damage.

    g. Arterial blood gases are likely to show respiratory alkalosis.

    h. If lactate is elevated, prognosis is poor.

    i. Check electrocardiogram (EKG).

    j. Check chest x-ray (CXR).

V. Treatment

    a. Remove patient from direct sunlight.

    b. Supportive measures

        i. May need to intubate.

        ii. Obtain IV access and provide IV dextrose and normal (or half-normal) saline.

    c. External cooling

        i. Goal is to lower core temperature to 38.8°C (101.8°F).

        ii. Evaporation techniques

            1. Remove clothing.

            2. Spray with cool water or wrap with wet towels.

        iii. Immersion techniques

            1. Use cooling blankets.

            2. Immerse in cold water or ice.

            3. Place ice packs over patient.

            4. Caveat—these techniques can cause the patient to shiver, thereby generating heat, so it is better to use evaporation method.

    d. Internal cooling

        i. Used when external techniques fail

        ii. Cold water irrigation to the stomach or rectum

        iii. Peritoneal lavage

        iv. Cardiopulmonary bypass

    e. Cooling should be stopped when core temperature reaches 38°C to 39°C (≈101°F) to avoid progressive hypothermia.

    f. Resume cooling if fever rebounds.

    g. What NOT to do:

        i. Do not give patient acetaminophen, aspirin, salt, or beverages containing alcohol or caffeine.

        ii. Do not rub alcohol on the skin.

VI. Prognosis

    a. With delayed treatment, mortality is 80%.

    b. With early treatment, mortality is 10%.

HEAT EXHAUSTION

I. Causes
   a. Occurs because of impaired or inadequate sweating.
   b. Occurs if a person is exerting him/herself in hot ambient temperature, and when he/she does not drink enough fluids to replace lost water and electrolytes.
II. Risk factors
   a. Similar to those of heatstroke.
III. Symptoms and signs
   a. General—malaise, fatigue, weakness, nausea, vomiting, and urge to defecate
   b. Neurologic—headache, dizziness, vertigo, and syncope
   c. Skin—pale, cool, and clammy
   d. Vital signs
      i. Core body temperature increases $>38°C$ (100.4°F) but remains $<40.5°C$ (104.9°F).
         1. The patient usually syncopizes before having had the chance to continue exertion.
         2. Therefore, the temperature does not continue to rise as it does in heatstroke.
      ii. Tachycardia
      iii. Hypotension
IV. Treatment
   a. If mild, may treat at home.
      i. Place patient in recumbent position, elevate legs.
      ii. Oral rehydration is with electrolyte-containing fluids (such as Gatorade).
   b. Recovery should occur within a few hours.
   c. If symptoms continue
      i. IV hydration with dextrose plus normal (or half normal) saline
      ii. More aggressive external cooling techniques
   d. Moderate to severe heat exhaustion can proceed to heatstroke.

LITHIUM-INDUCED NEUROTOXIC "SYNDROME"

NOTE:

There is no established, specific, one neurologic syndrome caused by lithium, labeled as such. And yet, for the reason that the neurologic sequelae of lithium excess can be devastating for the patients, some of whom may require total care if they survive, that we choose to make the psychiatrist aware of this here.

I. Lithium poses a special danger because lithium has a very narrow therapeutic index, that is, its therapeutic dose closely correlates with the dose that may produce a toxic reaction. Neurotoxic effects may also occur with therapeutic lithium levels.

II. Do not start lithium on patients before doing the prelithium work-up (see Appendix A).

III. Use caution when using lithium in the following conditions:

a. Renal insufficiency—lithium is excreted through the kidneys, and it can accumulate rapidly in the presence of renal insufficiency.

b. Dehydration—patients who develop polyuria from lithium are at a risk of toxicity secondary to dehydration from the decreased ability of kidneys to concentrate urine.

Dehydration also causes fluid and electrolyte imbalance.

c. Infections, fever—fever (Adityanjee, 2005) may be a precipitant to the development of neurotoxicity, and is also a manifestation of neurotoxicity.

Gastroenteritis can cause dehydration as well.

Note: Leukocytosis without underlying infection can occur in the acute phase of lithium toxicity.

d. Hyponatremia—patients who have low serum sodium levels, or patients who are on sodium restricted diet, or patients who take medications that decrease sodium levels (thiazide diuretics, furosemide, ethacrynic acid, angiotensin-converting enzyme [ACE] inhibitors) are candidates for lithium toxicity because lithium excretion depends on normal sodium concentrations. Low serum sodium encourages the kidneys to reabsorb more lithium ions.

e. Neurologic conditions—patients prone to seizures or who have other neurologic illnesses are candidates for lithium toxicity.

    f. Elderly patients—the elderly have a lower glomerular filtration rate and a lower creatinine clearance.
Their blood level of lithium may be high even if the given dose of lithium is small.

IV. Drug interactions with lithium
- a. ACE inhibitors decrease sodium levels.
- b. Thiazides diuretics, furosemide, and ethacrynic acid decrease sodium levels.
- c. Nonsteroidal anti-inflammatory drugs (NSAIDs) decrease lithium clearance, and thereby increase lithium levels.
- d. Certain antibiotics
  - i. Macrolides
  - ii. Antifungals (eg., metronidazole)
  - iii. Trimethoprim (one case report noted)
- e. Psychiatric medications
  - i. Selective serotonin reuptake inhibitors
    1. Interaction can either increase or decrease lithium levels.
    2. Lithium toxicity can be seen at normal lithium levels.
  - ii. Tricyclic antidepressants (TCAs)
    1. Because TCA and lithium can lower seizure threshold, there is the potential for an additive effect.
    2. Specifically, there is an increased risk of neurotoxicity.
  - iii. Antipsychotics
    1. Concomitant use can increase risk of extrapyramidal side effects.
       - a. Note—this phenomenon does NOT improve with anticholinergic medications.
    2. Increased risk of neuroleptic malignant syndrome.

V. Side effects of lithium by systems
- a. Gastrointestinal—nausea, vomiting, diarrhea
- b. Hematologic—leukocytosis
- c. Endocrine—hypothyroidism, hyperparathyroidism
- d. Renal—nephrogenic diabetes insipidus, renal failure
- e. Cardiac—arrhythmia, prolonged QT
- f. Neurologic—see subsequent text

VI. Neurologic consequences
- a. Predominate in most cases, especially moderate to severe cases.
- b. Central nervous system (CNS) is the primary target system for toxicity.
- c. May be fatal.
- d. Correlation between levels and symptoms
  - i. Serum level does not necessarily correlate with toxicity.
  - ii. Patients with high lithium levels may not have symptoms during the acute phase of intoxication because of delayed distribution of lithium.
  - iii. When levels decrease, patient may continue to have symptoms because lithium accumulates in white matter. Note

that cerebrospinal fluid (CSF) levels do not correlate with the level accumulated in white matter.

iv. With chronic intoxication, patient may be symptomatic at slightly elevated levels because, as lithium has already accumulated in the CNS, the system can not tolerate higher levels.

NOTE:

Both acute and chronic toxicity can occur within the therapeutic range.

VII. Symptoms/signs of neurotoxicity

NOTE:

Neurotoxicity may manifest as worsening psychosis.

---

  a. Mild
     i. Weakness
     ii. Fine or coarse tremor
     iii. drowsiness
     iv. Mild confusion
  b. Moderate
     i. Muscle fasciculation/twitching
     ii. Hyperreflexia
     iii. Significant confusion
     iv. Lethargy
     v. Dizziness
     vi. Vertigo
     vii. Nystagmus
     viii. Ataxia
     ix. Choreoathetosis
  c. Severe
     i. Myoclonus
     ii. Markedly increased deep tendon reflexes
     iii. Syncope
     iv. Coma
     v. Seizures
  d. Seizures and agitation can lead to hyperthermia and rhabdomyolysis
  e. Chronic effects
     i. Cerebellar dysfunction
        1. Dysarthria
        2. Scanning speech
        3. Nystagmus
        4. Truncal and limb ataxia
        5. Broad-based gait
     ii. Cognitive problems

1. Short-term memory impairment
2. Dementia (rarely occurs)

NOTE:

10% of patients are left with chronic neurologic consequences, as described in the preceding text.

VIII. Workup
   a. Check lithium level every 2 to 4 hours
   b. Blood urea nitrogen (BUN), creatinine
   c. Electrolytes
   d. Anion gap decreased
   e. Toxicology screen
   f. Electrocardiogram (EKG)
   g. CT head to rule out trauma and if severe neurologic consequences.
   h. Electroencephalogram (EEG) may show the following abnormalities:
      i. Diffuse slowing, nonspecific changes
      ii. "Runs of periodic sharp waves ... triphasic complexes ... widespread slow activity alternating with runs of periodic sharp waves," (Smith, 1988) which is similar to EEG seen in Creutzfelt-Jakob disease
      iii. "Increased theta and delta especially in frontal areas with triphasic waves and sharp waves in frontal areas." (Broussolle, 1989).

IX. Treatment
   a. Stop lithium
   b. Supportive care
   c. Gastric lavage if acute intoxication, and if the patient presents within 1 hour of an overdose
   d. Activated charcoal if there is a possibility of coingestion.
   e. Whole bowel irrigation if acute intoxication with sustained release
   f. Hydration with normal to half-normal saline
   g. Sodium polystyrene sulfonate (Kayexelate)
      i. Binds lithium and aids its elimination.
      ii. May result in hypokalemia and hypernatremia, so need to monitor fluid and electrolyte status.
      iii. Contraindicated if the patient has renal failure or congestive heart failure.
   h. Indications for dialysis
      i. Unstable presentation
      ii. Severe symptoms/signs
      iii. Renal failure
      iv. Consider dialysis if acute intoxication and lithium level >4 mEq per L

   v. Consider dialysis if chronic intoxication and lithium level
       >2 mEq per L
i. Therapy for long-term effects
   i. Cognitive rehabilitation
   ii. Physical rehabilitation

REMEMBER:

Lithium can cause severe toxicities involving multiple organs. Therefore, when given a choice, it is better to use another mood stabilizer such as valproate.

Monitoring for Psychiatric Medications

I. General
   a. In the medically ill, consideration needs to be given to
      i. The side effects of psychotropics
      ii. The effects of the medical illness on metabolism of psychotropics
   b. In those with liver disease, psychiatric medications should be carefully adjusted; monitor liver function tests (LFTs).
   c. In those presenting with depression, mania, psychosis, or a change in mental status, check basic laboratory tests.
      i. Rule out disorders due to a general medical condition as well as substance-induced disorders.
         1. Basic laboratory tests include a complete blood count (CBC), chemistry panel, LFTs, thyroid stimulating hormone (TSH), pregnancy test, and urine drug screen.
II. Atypical antipsychotics
   a. Monitoring protocols should take into account concern for metabolic disturbances, which tend to be worst with clozapine and olanzapine, and least with aripiprazole and ziprasidone. Periodically monitor weight, abdominal obesity, blood pressure, fasting blood glucose, and the lipid profile. Some psychiatrists may do this independently or in conjunction with the patient's primary care physician.
      i. If significant abnormalities are found (i.e., $\geq 5\%$ adverse change), consider switching to a different antipsychotic, behavioral modification (e.g., diet and exercise), and/or additional medical treatments.
   b. Special considerations
      i. Clozapine (Clozaril)
         1. Because of the risk of agranulocytosis (1%–2%), check a white blood cell (WBC) and differential count
            a. At baseline before the initiation of treatment
            b. Every week, for the first 6 months of therapy, and every 2 weeks thereafter
            c. Weekly for 4 weeks after discontinuation of clozapine
         2. If WBC <3k or granulocytes are <1.5k, stop clozapine
            a. Clozapine may be restarted after normalization of WBC if
               i. WBC was never <2k or granulocytes were never <1k
      ii. Patients with heart disease, a family history of sudden death, or those taking drugs that prolong the QTc

      1. An EKG should be checked due to the risk of conduction disturbances (e.g., prolonged QTc).

        a. Ziprasidone (Geodon), in particular, carries an Food and Drug Administration (FDA) warning regarding prolonged QTc; however, the effect is rarely of clinical significance.

   iii. Quetiapine (Seroquel)

      1. "The emergence of cataracts in toxicology studies of dogs has unclear, if any, implications for human use; although the current U.S. label advise baseline and subsequent 6-month slit-lamp examinations, there is no evidence that cataracts occur in relation to the drug in humans." (Rosenbaum, 2005).

III. Mood stabilizers

   a. Carbamazepine (Tegretol)

     i. Monitoring protocol (see Table A.1)

TABLE A.1 Monitoring Protocol for Carbamazepine

Tests	When to Check?
Carbamazepine level (check 12 hr after the last dose)	At baseline, twice a week while titrating dose, monthly for 3 mo, then semiannually (therapeutic level = 8–12 μg/mL)
Free carbamazepine level (check 12 hr after the last dose)	Check along with carbamazepine level when the patient is on multiple agents that interfere with protein binding
CBC and differential (to check for agranulocytosis, leukopenia, and thrombocytopenia)	At baseline, every 2 wk for the first 2 mo, and thereafter once every 3 mo
Liver function tests	At baseline, every 4 wk for the first 2 mo, and thereafter once every 3 mo
Basic chemistry panel (hyponatremia can be a side effect)	At baseline, 1 wk, 1 mo, and then semiannually
EKG (to check for conduction disturbances)	At baseline and yearly
Pregnancy test (carbamazepine is category D)	At baseline and monthly in non-compliant patients

CBC, complete blood count; EKG, electrocardiogram.

NOTE:

FDA category D medications are teratogenic, and yet may be used during pregnancy if the benefits outweigh the potential risks; clear and open discussion with the patient is imperative.

  b. Oxcarbazepine (Trileptal)
      i. Monitoring protocol (see Table A.2)

TABLE A.2 Monitoring Protocol for Oxcarbazepine

Tests	When to Check?
Oxcarbazepine level	There is NO established blood level
Liver function tests	At baseline, 1 wk, 1 mo, and then semiannually
Basic chemistry panel (for electrolytes, BUN, and creatinine)	At baseline, 1 wk, 1 mo, and then semiannually
Pregnancy test (oxcarbazepine is category D)	At baseline and monthly in noncompliant patients

BUN, blood urea nitrogen.

  c. Lithium
      i. Monitoring protocol (see Table A.3)

TABLE A.3 Monitoring Protocol for Lithium

Tests	When to Check?
Lithium level (check 12 hr after the last dose)	At baseline, twice a week while titrating dose, and semiannually (maintenance level = 0.6–1.2 mEq/L)
Basic chemistry (for electrolytes, BUN, creatinine)	At baseline, twice a week while titrating dose, 1 mo later, and then semiannually
Urinalysis	At baseline, at 3 months, and semiannually
Thyroid function tests (TSH reflex)	At baseline and yearly
Pregnancy test (lithium is category D)	At baseline and monthly in noncompliant patients
EKG (to check for conduction disturbances)	At baseline and routinely, if indicated
CBC (to check for leukocytosis)	At baseline and routinely, if indicated

BUN, blood urea nitrogen, TSH, thyroid stimulating hormone; EKG, electrocardiogram; CBC, complete blood count.

  d. Valproic acid (Depakote, Depakene, Divalproex)
      i. Monitoring protocol (see Table A.4)
IV. Stimulants
  a. An EKG is not necessarily needed for a young, healthy patient; however, sudden death has been reported in those with cardiac abnormalities; use clinical judgment and obtain baseline and routine EKGs if there is any question.

TABLE A.4 Monitoring Protocol for Valproic Acid

Tests	When to Check?
Valproate level (check 12 hr after the last dose)	At baseline, twice a week while titrating dose, 1 mo later, 3 mo later, and semiannually (therapeutic level = 50–120 μg/mL)
Free valproate level (check 12 hr after the last dose)	Check along with valproate level when the patient is on multiple agents that interfere with protein binding
Basic chemistry (for electrolytes)	At baseline and semiannually
Liver function tests	At baseline and semiannually
CBC (to check for pancytopenia)	At baseline and semiannually
Pregnancy test (valproic acid is category D)	At baseline and monthly in noncompliant patients

CBC, complete blood count.

    b. Monitor blood pressure, heart rate, and weight loss in all patients routinely.

V. Selective serotonin reuptake inhibitors (SSRIs)

    a. Monitoring protocols—no specific laboratory monitoring is required.

VI. Tricyclic antidepressants (TCAs)

    a. An electrocardiogram (EKG) should be taken at baseline and during ongoing care to assess for conduction disturbances.

    b. Levels should be checked routinely, particularly in those who are elderly, have a poor response, or are high-risk individuals (see Table A.5).

TABLE A.5 Monitoring Tricyclic Antidepressant Blood Levels

	Therapeutic Level 12 Hours After the Last Dose (ng/mL)
Imipramine	200–250
Desipramine	125–150
Amitriptyline	75–175
Nortriptyline	50–150

REMEMBER:

Imipramine is converted to desipramine, so when checking imipramine levels, also check desipramine levels; likewise, amitriptyline is converted to nortriptyline, so when checking amitriptyline levels, also check nortriptyline levels.

Abbreviations

d	deci 10^{-1}
c	centi 10^{-2}
m	milli 10^{-3}
μ	micro 10^{-6}
n	nano 10^{-9}
p	pico 10^{-12}
f	femto 10^{-15}
a	atto 10^{-18}
α	alpha
β	beta
κ	kappa
μ	mu
$\downarrow$	decrease
$\uparrow$	increase
♀	male
♂	female
>	greater than
$\geq$	greater than or equal to
<	less than
$\leq$	less than or equal to
~	approximately
=	equals
$\pm$	with or without
ABCs	airway, breathing, circulation
ABG	arterial blood gas
ABI	ankle-brachial index
ACA	anterior cerebral artery
ACE-I	angiotensin-converting enzyme inhibitor
AG	anion gap
AIDS	acquired immunodeficiency syndrome
APTT	activated partial thromboplastin time
ARB	angiotension receptor blocker
AV	atriovenous
BID	twice a day
BM	bowel movement
BP	blood pressure
BPH	benign prostatic hypertrophy
bpm	beats per minute
BS	blood sugar
BUN	blood urea nitrogen
°C	degree Celsius
Ca	calcium
CAD	coronary artery disease
CAP	community acquired pneumonia
CBC	complete blood count

CCB	calcium channel blocker
CD4	helper T cells
CD8	suppressor T cells
CFU	colony forming unit
CHD	coronary heart disease
Chem-7	chemistry panel (includes Na, K, Cl, HCO_3, BUN, Cr, and BS)
CHF	congestive heart failure
CK, CPK	creatine kinase
Cl	chloride
CNS	central nervous system
COPD	chronic obstructive pulmonary disease
Cr	creatinine
CT/CAT scan	computed tomography
cTnI	cardiac troponin-I
CV	cardiovascular
CVD	cerebrovascular disease
CXR	chest x-ray
DBP	diastolic blood pressure
DIC	disseminated intravascular coagulopathy
DKA	diabetic ketoacidosis
dL	deciliter (100 mL)
DM	diabetes mellitus (at the pharmacy, DM = dextromethorphan)
DWI	diffusion-weighted imaging
EEG	electroencephalography
e.g.	for example
EGD	esophagogastroduodenoscopy
EKG	electrocardiogram
ELISA	enzyme linked immunosorbent assay
EMS	emergency medical services
EPS	extrapyramidal symptoms
ER	emergency room, extended release if referring to medication
etc.	et cetera
°F	degrees Fahrenheit
FDA	Food and Drug Administration
FEV_1	forced expiratory volume in 1 second
FPG	fasting plasma glucose
FTA ABS	fluorescent treponemal antibody absorption test
g	gram
GERD	gastroesophageal reflux disease
GFR	glomerular filtration rate
GI	gastrointestinal
GNR	gram negative rods
gtt	drops (or drip when associated with IV gtt)
HCO_3	bicarbonate
Hct	hematocrit
HDL	high density lipoprotein (good cholesterol)
Hg A_{1c}	glycated (glycosylated) hemoglobin
HgB/Hb	hemoglobin
HIV	human immunodeficiency virus
HR	heart rate
hr	hour
HSV	herpes simplex virus
HTN	hypertension
ICP	intracranial pressure

ICU	intensive care unit
i.e.	that is
IFG	impaired fasting glucose
Ig	immunoglobulin
IM	intramuscular
INR	international normalized ratio
IOP	intraocular pressure
IU	international unit
IUD	intrauterine device
IV	intravenous
K	potassium
k	1,000
kcal	kilocalorie
kg	kilogram
KOH	potassium hydroxide
L	liter
LDH	lactate dehydrogenase
LDL	low density lipoprotein (bad cholesterol)
LFTs	liver function tests
LP	lumbar puncture
LVH	left ventricular hypertrophy
MAOI	monoamine oxidase inhibitor
MAP	mean arterial pressure
MCA	middle cerebral artery
μg	microgram
MCH	mean corpuscular hemoglobin
MCHC	mean corpuscular hemoglobin
MCV	mean corpuscular volume
MDI	metered dose inhaler
mEq	milliequivalent
Mg	magnesium
mg	milligram
MI	myocardial infarction
min	minute
mL	milliliter
mm^3	cubic millimeter
mm Hg	millimeters of mercury
mmol	millimole
mol, mole	amount of a substance
mo	month
mOsm	milliosmols
MPV	mean platelet volume
MRA	magnetic resonance angiogram
MRI	magnetic resonance imaging
MRSA	methicillin-resistant *Staphylococcus aureus*
MS	multiple sclerosis
Na	sodium
N/A	not applicable
ng	nanogram
NPH	normal pressure hydrocephalus
NPH (Insulin)	neutral protamine hagedorn
NSAID	nonsteroidal anti-inflammatory drug
O_2	oxygen
OAB	overactive bladder

OCP	oral contraceptive pill
OD	oculus dexter (right eye)
ODT	oral disintegrating tablet
OGTT	oral glucose tolerance test
OS	oculus sinister (left eye)
OSA	obstructive sleep apnea
osm	osmolality, refers to the amount of solutes in a liquid
PAD	peripheral arterial disease
Pao_2	partial pressure of arterial oxygen
PCA	patient controlled analgesia
Pco_2	partial pressure of carbon dioxide
PCP	primary care physician
PEF	peak expiratory flow
PFTs	pulmonary function tests
PID	pelvic inflammatory disease
PO	by mouth (oral)
PPI	proton pump inhibitor
PR	by rectum
p.r.n	as needed
PT	prothrombin time
PT–INR	prothrombin time, international normalized ratio
PTT	partial thromboplastin time
PUD	peptic ulcer disease
PV	per vaginum
PVR	postvoid residual
q	every
qAC	before meals
qhs	at bedtime
QID	four times a day
qxh	every $\underline{x}$ hour (where $\underline{x}$ equals a number)
RBC	red blood cell
RDW	red cell distribution width
RPR	rapid plasma reagin (test for syphilis)
RR	respiratory rate
RUQ	right upper quadrant
SA	surface area
SAH	subarachnoid hemorrhage
SAo_2	arterial oxygen saturation
SBP	systolic blood pressure
SC	subcutaneous
SIADH	syndrome of inappropriate antidiuretic hormone secretion
SL	sublingual
SNRI	serotonin-norepinephrine reuptake inhibitor
SOB	shortness of breath
SR	sustained release
SSRI	selective serotonin reuptake inhibitor
STD	sexually transmitted disease
T_4	thyroxine
TCA	tricyclic antidepressant
Td	tetanus and diphtheria toxoids vaccination
TG	triglyceride
TIA	transient ischemic attack
TID	three times a day
TM	tympanic membrane

tPA	tissue plasminogen activator
TPO	thyroperoxidase
TSH	thyroid stimulating hormone
TURP	transurethral resection of the prostate
US	United States
UTI	urinary tract infection
UV	ultraviolet
VDRL	venereal disease research laboratory test
WBC	white blood cell
wk	week

BIBLIOGRAPHY

SECTION 1

American Diabetes Association: *Clinical Practice Recommendations 2004*. Diabetes Care, Jan 2004, Supplement 1.

Andreoli T, ed. *Cecil essentials of medicine*, 5th ed. Philadelphia: WB Saunders; 2001.

Bakerman P, Strausbauch P. *Bakerman's ABC's of interpretive laboratory data*, 3rd ed. Myrtle Beach: Interpretive Laboratory Data; 1994.

Fischbach FT, Dunning MB III, eds. *A manual of laboratory and diagnostic tests*, 7th ed. Philadelphia: Lippincott Williams & Wilkins; 2004.

Howanitz J, Howanitz P, eds. *Laboratory medicine, test selection and interpretation*. New York: Churchill Livingstone; 1991.

Kee JL. *Laboratory and diagnostic tests with nursing implicatons*, 7th ed. Upper Saddle River: Prentice Hall; 2005.

Krupp MA, Chatton MJ. *Current medical diagnosis and treatment*. Los Altos: Appleton & Lange; 1974.

Noe DA, Rock RC, eds. *Laboratory medicine, the selection and interpretation of clinical laboratory studies*. Philadelphia: Williams & Wilkins; 1994.

Tierney LM Jr, McPhee SJ, Papadakis MA, eds. *Current medical diagnosis and treatment*, 43rd ed. New York: Appleton & Lange/McGraw-Hill; 2004.

SECTION 2

2.1. Acetaminophen (APAP/Tylenol) Overdose

Bartlett D. Acetaminophen toxicity. *J Emerg Nurs*. 2004;30:281–283.

Rowden AK, Norvell J, Eldridge DL, et al. Acetaminophen Poisoning. *Clin Lab Med*. 2006;26:49–65.

Rumack BH, Matthew H. Acetaminophen poisoning and toxicity. *Pediatrics*. 1975;55(6):871–876.

2.2. Allergic Rhinitis (Allergies)

Greiner AN. Allergic rhinitis: Impact of the disease and considerations for management. *Med Clin North Am*. 2006;90:17–38.

2.3. Anaphylaxis

Lima MT, Marshall GD. Anaphylaxis and Serum Sickness. In: Rakel RE, Bope ET, eds. *Conn's current therapy*. Philadelphia: WB Saunders; 2006:915–917.

Scarlet C. Anaphylaxis. *J Infus Nurs*. 2006;29(1):39–44.

2.4. Anemia

Duffy TP. Microcytic and hypochromic anemias. In: Goldman L, Ausiello D, eds. *Cecil textbook of medicine*, 22nd ed. Philadelphia: WB Saunders; 2004:1003–1008.

Little DR. Ambulatory management of common forms of anemia. *Am Fam Physician*. 1999;59(6):1598–1606.

Stabler SP, Allen RH. Megaloblastic anemias. In: Goldman L, Ausiello D, eds. *Cecil textbook of medicine*, 22nd ed. Philadelphia: WB Saunders; 2004:1050–1057.

Zuckerman KS. Approach to the anemias. In: Goldman L, Ausiello D, eds. *Cecil textbook of medicine*, 22nd ed. Philadelphia: WB Saunders; 2004:963–971.

2.5. Angina

Lee TH, Goldman L. Evaluation of the patient with acute chest pain. *N Engl J Med*. 2000;342(16):1187–1195.

Mehta SB, Wu WC. Management of coronary heart disease: Stable angina, acute coronary syndrome, myocardial infarction. *Prim Care*. 2005;32:1057–1081.

Pozner CN, Levine M, Zane R. The cardiovascular effects of cocaine. *J Emerg Med*. 2005;29(2):173–178.

2.6. Antibiotic Cross-Sensitivities

Depta JPH, Pichler WJ. Cross-reactivity with drugs at the T cell level. *Curr Opin Allergy Clin Immunol*. 2003;3:261–267.

Gruchalla RS, Pirmohamed M. Antibiotic allergy. *N Engl J Med*. 2006;354: 601–609.

Park MA, Li JTC. Diagnosis and management of penicillin allergy. *Mayo Clin Proc*. 2005;80(3):405–410.

2.7. Aphthous Ulcers (Canker Sores)

Hanly JG, Fisk JD, McCurdy G, et al. Neuropsychiatric syndromes in patients with systemic lupus erythematosus and rheumatoid arthritis. *J Rheumatol*. 2005;32(8):1459–1466.

McBride DR. Management of aphthous ulcers. *Am Fam Physician*. 2000; 62(1):149–154, 160.

Nkam I, Cottereau MJ. Acute psychosis and Behcet's disease: A case report. *Encephale*. 2006;32(3 Pt 1):385–388.

2.8. Arrhythmias

Akhtar M. Chapter 59–Cardiac arrhythmias with supraventricular origin. *Goldman: Cecil textbook of medicine*, 22nd ed. WB Saunders; 319–327.

Delacrétaz E. Supraventricular tachycardia. *N Engl J Med*. 2006;354(10): 1039–1051.

Gage BF, Waterman AD, Shannon W, et al. Validation of clinical classification schemes for predicting stroke: Results from the national registry of atrial fibrillation. *JAMA*. 2001;285(22):2864–2870.

Hebbar AK, Hueston WJ. Management of common arrhythmias: Part I. Supraventricular arrhythmias. *Am Fam Physician*. 2002;65(12):2479–2486.

Hebbar AK, Hueston WJ. Management of common arrhythmias: Part II. Ventricular arrhythmias and arrhythmias in special populations. *Am Fam Physician*. 2002;65(12):2491–2496.

2.9. Asthma

Brown ES, Chandler PA. Mood and cognitive changes during systemic corticosteroid therapy. *Prim Care Companion J Clin Psychiatry*. 2001; 3(1):17–21.

Brown ES, Khan DA, Nejtek VA. The psychiatric side effects of corticosteroids. *Ann Allergy Asthma Immunol*. 1999;83(6 Pt 1):495–503.

Mackay IR, Rosen FS. Asthma. *N Engl J Med*. 2001;344(5):350–362.

National Asthma Education and Prevention Program. Expert panel report: Guidelines for the diagnosis and management of asthma update on selected topics–2002. *J Allergy Clin Immunol*. 2002;110:S141–S219.

Naureckas ET, Solway J. Mild asthma. *N Engl J Med*. 2001;345(17):1257–1262.

2.10. Bronchitis (Acute)

Knutson D, Braun C. Diagnosis and management of acute bronchitis. *Am Fam Physician*. 2002;65(10):2039–2044.

Linder JA. Acute bronchitis. In: Rakel RE, Bope ET, eds. *Conn's current therapy 2006*. Philadelphia: WB Saunders; 2006:319–321.

Linder JA, Sim I. Antibiotic treatment of acute bronchitis in smokers. *J Gen Intern Med*. 2002;17:230–234.

2.11. Burns

Johnson RM, Richard R. Partial-thickness burns: Identification and management. *Adv Skin Wound Care*. 2003;16:178–189.

Morgan ED, Bledsoe SC, Barker J. Ambulatory management of burns. *Am Fam Physician*. 2000;62(9):2015–2029.

2.12. Candidiasis–Mucocutaneous Infections

Akpan A, Morgan R. Oral Candidiasis. *Postgrad Med J*. 2002;78:455–459.

Kauffman CA. Candidiasis. In: Goldman L, Ausiello D, eds. *Cecil textbook of medicine*, 22nd ed. Philadelphia: WB Saunders; 2004:2053–2056.

2.13. Cerebrovascular Disease: Transient Ischemic Attack and Stroke

Ferri FF. Stroke. In: Ferri FF, ed. *Ferri: Practical guide to the care of the medical patient*, 6th ed. St. Louis: Mosby; 2004:725–739.

Solenski NJ. Transient ischemic attacks: Part I. Diagnosis and evaluation. *Am Fam Physician*. 2004;69(7):1665–1674, 1679–1680.

Solenski NJ. Transient ischemic attacks: Part II. Treatment. *Am Fam Physician*. 2004;69(7):1681–1688.

2.14. Chronic Obstructive Pulmonary Disease

Hunter MH, King DE. COPD: Management of acute exacerbations and chronic stable disease. *Am Fam Physician*. 2001;64(4):603–612.

Sutherland ER, Cherniack RM. Management of chronic obstructive pulmonary disease. *N Engl J Med*. 2004;350(26):2689–2697.

2.15. The Common Cold

Heikkinen T, Järvinen A. The common cold. *Lancet*. 2003;361:51–59.

Lorber B. The common cold [Perspective]. *J Gen Intern Med*. 1996;11(4):229–236.

2.16. Congestive Heart Failure

DeWitt CR, Waksman JC. Pharmacology, pathophysiology and management of calcium channel blocker and beta-blocker toxicity. *Toxicol Rev*. 2004;23(4):223–238.

Jessup M, Brozena S. Medical progress: Heart failure. *N Engl J Med*. 2003;348(20):2007–2018.

Olson, KR. Poisoning. *Current medical diagnosis and treatment 2004*, 43rd ed. McGraw-Hill; 2004:1559–1560.

Silver MA. Heart failure. In: Rakel RE, Bope ET, eds. *Conn's current therapy 2006*. Philadelphia: WB Saunders; 2006:409–414.

2.17. Conjunctivitis (Acute)

Katz SE, Kopp AM. Conjunctivitis. In: Rakel RE, Bope ET, eds. *Conn's current therapy 2006*. Philadelphia: WB Saunders; 2006:230–233.

2.18. Constipation (Chronic)

Arce DA, Ermocilla CA, Costa H. Evaluation of constipation. *Am Fam Physician*. 2002;65(11):2283–2290.

Bleser S, Brunton S, Carmichael B, et al. Management of chronic constipation: Recommendations from a consensus panel. *J Fam Pract*. 2005;54(8):691–698.

Lembo A, Camilleri M. Chronic constipation. *N Engl J Med*. 2003;349(14):1360–1368.

Mason HJ, Serrano-Ikkos E, Kamm MA. Psychological morbidity in women with idiopathic constipation. *Am J Gastroenterol*. 2000;95(10):2852–2857.

2.19. Cough

Holmes RL, Fadden CT. Evaluation of the patient with chronic cough. *Am Fam Physician*. 2004;69(9):2159–2166, 2169.

Irwin RS, Madison JM. The diagnosis and treatment of cough. *N Engl J Med*. 2000;343(23):1715–1721.

2.20. Dental Procedures in Patients at Risk (Prophylaxis)

Dajani AS, Taubert KA, Wilson W, et al. Prevention of bacterial endo-carditis: Recommendations by the American Heart Association. *Clin Infect Dis.* 1997;25:1448–1458.

2.21. Diabetes Mellitus

Ajilore O, Haroon E, Kumaran S, et al. *Measurement of Brain Metabo-lites in Patients with type 2 Diabetes and Major Depression Using Proton Magnetic Resonance Spectroscopy.* Neuropsychopharmacology advance online publication 20 Dec. 2006.

American Diabetic Association. *Clinical Practice Recommendations 2004,* Diabetic Care, Jan 2004, Supplement 1.

Aronne LJ, Segal KR. Weight gain in the treatment of mood disorders. *J Clin Psychiatry.* 2003;64(Suppl 8):22–29.

Daneman D. Type 1 Diabetes. *Lancet.* 2006;367:847–858.

Ferri FF. Endocrinology. In: Ferri FF, ed. *Ferri: Practical guide to the care of the medical patient,* 6th ed. St. Louis: Mosby; 2004:267–291.

Ganguli R. Weight gain associated with antipsychotic drugs. *J Clin Psychi-atry.* 1999;60(Suppl 21):20–24.

Katon W, Lin EH, Kroenke K, et al. The association of depression and anxiety with medical symptom burden in patients with chronic med-ical illness. *Gen Hosp Psychiatry.* 2007;29(2):147–155.

Mirza SA. Diabetes mellitus in adults. In: Rakel RE, Bope ET, eds. *Conn's current therapy 2006.* Philadelphia: WB Saunders; 2006:701–708.

Nathan DM. Initial management of glycemia in type 2 diabetes mellitus. *N Engl J Med.* 2002;347(17):1342–1349.

Stumvoll M, Goldstein BJ, van Haeften TW. Type 2 Diabetes: Principles of pathogenesis and therapy. *Lancet.* 2005;365:1333–1346.

2.22. Diarrhea

Faresjo A, Grodzinsky E, Johansson S, et al. A population-based case-control study of work and psychosocial problems in patients with irritable bowel syndrome–women are more seriously affected than men. *Am J Gastroenterol.* 2007;102(2):371–379.

Henningsen P, Zimmermann T, Sattel H. Medically unexplained phys-ical symptoms, anxiety, and depression: A meta-analytic review. *Psychosom Med.* 2003;65(4):528–533.

Labus JS, Mayer EA, Chang L, et al. The central role of gastrointestinal-specific anxiety in irritable bowel syndrome: Further validation of the visceral sensitivity index. *Psychosom Med.* 2007;69(1):89–98.

Schiller LR. Chronic Diarrhea. *Gastroenterology.* 2004;127:287–293.

Semrad CE, Powell DW. Approach to the patient with diarrhea and mal-absorption. In: Goldman L, Ausiello D, eds. *Cecil textbook of medicine,* 22nd ed. Philadelphia: WB Saunders; 2004:842–860.

2.23. Dysmenorrhea (Menstrual Cramps)

Durain D. Primary dysmenorrhea: Assessment and management update. *J Midwifery Womens Health.* 2004;49:520–528.

French L. Dysmenorrhea. *Am Fam Physician*. 2005;71(2):285–292.

2.24. Dyspepsia

Dickerson LM, King DE. Evaluation and management of nonulcer dyspepsia. *Am Fam Physician*. 2004;70(1):107–114.

Fisher RS, Parkman HP. Management of nonulcer dyspepsia. *N Engl J Med*. 1998;339(19):1376–1381.

2.25. Ear Ailments

Pichichero ME. Acute otitis media: Part I. Improving diagnostic accuracy. *Am Fam Physician*. 2000;61(7):2051–2056.

Pichichero ME. Acute otitis media: Part II. Treatment in an era of increasing antibiotic resistance. *Am Fam Physician*. 2000;61(8):2410–2416.

Sander R. Otitis externa: A practical guide to treatment and prevention. *Am Fam Physician*. 2001;63(5):927–936, 941–942.

2.26. Epilepsy

Alsaadi TM, Marquez AV. Psychogenic nonepileptic seizures. *Am Fam Physician*. 2005;72(5):849–856.

Browne TR, Holmes GL. Epilepsy. *N Engl J Med*. 2001;344(15):1145–1151.

LaFrance WC Jr, Barry JJ. Update on treatments of psychological nonepileptic seizures. *Epilepsy Behav*. 2005;7(3):364–374.

Sirven JI, Waterhouse E. Management of Status Epilepticus. *Am Fam Physician*. 2003;68(3):469–476.

2.27. Epistaxis (Nosebleed)

Kucik CJ, Clenney T. Management of epistaxis. *Am Fam Physician*. 2005;71(2):305–311, 312.

Pope LER, Hobbs CGL. Epistaxis: An update on current management. *Postgrad Med J*. 2005;81:309–314.

2.28. Foot Ailments

Ferri FF. Tinea pedis. In: Ferri FF, ed. *Ferri: Ferri's clinical advisor: Instant diagnosis and treatment*, 8th ed. Philadelphia: Mosby; 2006:846, 910–911.

Mikolich D. *Onychomycosis. Ferri: Ferri: Ferri's clinical advisor: Instant diagnosis and treatment*, 8th ed. Philadelphia: Mosby; 2006:588–589.

2.29. Gastroesophageal Reflux Disease

Heidelbaugh JJ, Nostrant TT, Kim C, et al. Management of gastroesophageal reflux disease. *Am Fam Physician*. 2003;68(7):1311–1318, 1321–1322.

2.30. Glaucoma, Open-Angle

Alward WLM. Medical Management of Glaucoma. *N Engl J Med*. 1998;339(18):1298–1307.

Distelhorst JS, Hughes GM. Open-angle glaucoma. *Am Fam Physician*. 2003;67(9):1937–1944, 1950.

2.31. Gout

Akhondzadeh S, Milajerdi MR, Amini H, et al. Allopurinol as an adjunct to lithium and haloperidol for treatment of patients with acute mania: A double-blind, randomized, placebo-controlled trial. *Bipolar Disord*. 2006;8:485–489.

Buie LW, Oertel MD, Cala SO, et al. Allopurinol as adjuvant therapy in poorly responsive or treatment refractory schizophrenia. *Ann Pharmacother*. 2006;40(12):2200–2204.

Clunie M, Crone LA, Klassen L, et al. Psychiatric side effects of in-domethacin in parturients. *Can J Anaesth*. 2003;50(6):586–588.

Lara DR, Belmonte-de-Abreu P, Souza DO. Allopurinol for refractory aggression and self-inflicted behaviour. *J Psychopharmacol*. 2000;14(1): 81–83.

Lara DR, Cruz MR, Xavier F, et al. Allopurinol for the treatment of ag-gressive behaviour in patients with dementia. *Int Clin Psychopharmacol*. 2003;18(1):53–55.

Suresh E. Diagnosis and management of gout: A rational approach. *Postgrad Med J*. 2005;81:572–579.

Terkeltaub RA. Gout. *N Engl J Med*. 2003;349(17):1647–1655.

Tharumaratnam D, Bashford S, Khan SA. Indomethacin induced psy-chosis. *Postgrad Med J*. 2000;76(901):736–737.

2.32. Headaches (Cephalalgia)

Bair MJ, Robinson RL, Katon W, et al. Depression and pain comorbidity: A literature review. *Arch Intern Med*. 2003;163(20):2433–2445.

Clinch CR. Evaluation of acute headaches in adults. *Am Fam Physician*. 2001;63(4):685–692.

Dodick DW. Chronic daily headache. *N Engl J Med*. 2006;354(2):158–165.

Fava M, Mallinckrodt CH, Detke MJ, et al. The effect of duloxetine on painful physical symptoms in depressed patients: Do improvements in these symptoms result in higher remission rates? *J Clin Psychiatry*. 2004;65(4):521–530.

Gallagher RM. Headache. In: Rakel RE, Bope ET, eds. *Conn's current therapy 2006*. Philadelphia: WB Saunders; 2006:1118–1124.

Goadsby PJ, Lipton RB, Ferrari MD. Migraine–Current understanding and treatment. *N Engl J Med*. 2002;346(4):257–270.

Maizels M. The patient with daily headaches. *Am Fam Physician*. 2004; 70(12):2299–2306, 2313–2314.

USP DI (United States Pharmacopeia Dispensing Information) Editorial Group. *UspDi Vol 1, Drug Information for the Health Care Professional, 24th Ed*. Greenwood Village: Thomson Micromedex, 2004.

2.33. Hemorrhoids

Alonso-Coelle P, Castillejo MM. Office evaluation and treatment of hem-orrhoids. *J Fam Pract*. 2003;52(5):366–374.

Pfenninger JL, Zainea GG. Common anorectal conditions: Part II. Lesions. *Am Fam Physician*. 2001;64(1):77–88.

Vrees MD, Weiss EG. Hemorrhoids, anal fissure, anorectal abscess, and fistula. In: Rakel RE, Bope ET, eds. *Conn's current therapy 2006*. Philadelphia: WB Saunders; 2006:639–641.

2.34. Herpes Simplex Virus (HSV)

Kimberlin DW, Rouse DJ. Genital herpes. *N Engl J Med*. 2004;350(19): 1970–1977.

Whitley RJ. Herpes simplex virus infections. In: Goldman L, Ausiello D, eds. *Cecil textbook of medicine*, 22nd ed. Philadelphia: WB Saunders; 2004; 1989–1992.

Whitley RJ, Roizman B. Herpes simplex virus infections. *Lancet*. 2001; 357:1513–1518.

2.35. Hyperlipidemia

Safeer RS, Ugalat PS. Cholesterol treatment guidelines update. *Am Fam Physician*. 2002;65(5):871–880.

2.36. Hypertension (Essential/Primary)

August P. Initial treatment of hypertension. *N Engl J Med*. 2003;348(7): 610–617.

Miller ER, Jehn ML. New high blood pressure guidelines create new at-risk classification. *J Cardiovasc Nurs*. 2004;19(6):367–371.

Onusko E. Diagnosing secondary hypertension. *Am Fam Physician*. 2003; 67(1):67–74.

Price WA, Giannini AJ. Neurotoxicity caused by lithium-verapamil synergism. *J Clin Pharmacol*. 1986;26:717.

The Sixth Report of the Joint National Committee on Prevention, Detection, evaluation, and treatment of high blood pressure. *Arch Intern Med*. 1997;157:2413–2446. [Erratum: *Arch Intern Med*. 1998;158:573.]

2.37. Hyperkalemia

Kokko JP. Fluids and electrolytes: Disturbances of potassium balance. In: Goldman L, Ausiello D, eds. *Cecil textbook of medicine*, 22nd ed. Philadelphia: Saunders; 2004; 669–687.

Rastergar A, Soleimani M. Hypokalaemia and hyperkalaemia. *Postgrad Med J*. 2001;77:759–764.

2.38. Hypokalemia

Kokko JP. Fluids and electrolytes. In: Goldman L, Ausiello D, eds. *Cecil textbook of medicine*, 22nd ed. Philadelphia: WB Saunders; 2004; 669–687.

Rastergar A, Soleimani M. Hypokalaemia and hyperkalaemia. *Postgrad Med J*. 2001;77:759–764.

2.39. Hypothyroidism

Bocchetta A, Loviselli A. Lithium treatment and thyroid abnormalities. *Clin Pract Epidemol Ment Health*. 2006;2:23.

Bokhari R, Bhatara VS, Bandettini F, et al. Postpartum psychosis and postpartum thyroiditis. *Psychoneuroendocrinology.* 1998;23(6):643–650.

Davis JD, Stern RA, Flashman LA. Cognitive and neuropsychiatric aspects of subclinical hypothyroidism: Significance in the elderly. *Curr Psychiatry Rep.* 2003;5(5):384–390.

Ferri FF. Endocrinology. In: Ferri FF, ed. *Ferri: Practical guide to the care of the medical patient*, 6th ed. St. Louis: Mosby; 2004; 317–319.

Nierenberg AA, Fava M, Trivedi MH, et al. A comparison of lithium and T(3) augmentation following two failed medication treatments for depression: A STAR*D report. *Am J Psychiatry.* 2006;163(9): 1519–1530.

Singer PA. Hypothyroidism. In: Rakel RE, Bope ET, eds. *Conn's current therapy 2006*. Philadelphia: WB Saunders; 2006:802–806.

2.40. Influenza

Couch RB. Prevention and treatment of influenza. *N Engl J Med.* 2000; 343(24):1778–1787.

Eccles R. Understanding the symptoms of the common cold and influenza. *Lancet Infect Dis.* 2005;5(11):718–725.

Mouton CP, Bazaldua OV, Pierce B, et al. Common infections in older adults. *Am Fam Physician.* 2001;63(2):257–268.

2.41. Menopause

Cutson TM, Meuleman E. Managing Menopause. *Am Fam Physician.* 2000;61:1391–1400, 1405–1406.

Manson JE, Martin KA. Postmenopausal hormone-replacement therapy. *N Engl J Med.* 2001;345(1):34–40.

Shifren JL, Schiff I. Menopause. In: Rakel RE, Bope ET, eds. *Conn's current therapy 2006*. Philadelphia: WB Saunders; 2006:1300–1334.

2.42. Nausea/Vomiting

Jordan K, Schmoll HJ, Aapro MS. Comparative activity of antiemetic drugs. *Crit Rev Oncol Hematol.* 2007;61(2):162–175.

Miser WF. Nausea and Vomiting. In: Rakel RE, Bope ET, eds. *Conn's current therapy*. Philadelphia: WB Saunders; 2006:5–10.

2.43. Osteoporosis (Postmenopausal)

Rosen CJ. Postmenopausal osteoporosis. *N Engl J Med.* 2005;353(6):595–603.

Shifren JL, Schiff I. *Menopause. Rakel: Conn's current therapy 2006*. 58th ed. WB Saunders; 2006;1300–1303.

World Health Organization. *Assessment of fracture risk and its application to screening for postmenopausal osteoporosis*. Technical report series. Geneva: WHO: 1994; 843.

2.44. Pain

Douglass AB. Section 1–Symptomatic care pending diagnosis: Pain. In: Rakel RE, Bope ET, eds. *Conn's current therapy 2006*. Philadelphia: WB Saunders; 2006:1–5.

Max MB. Pain. In: Goldman L, Ausiello D, eds. *Cecil textbook of medicine*, 22nd ed. Philadelphia: WB Saunders; 2004;138–145.

USP DI (United States Pharmacopeia Dispensing Information) Editorial Group. *USP DI Vol 1, Drug information for the health care professional*, 24th ed. Greenwood Village: Thomson Micromedex, 2004.

2.45. Peptic Ulcer Disease

Saad RJ, Scheiman JM. Diagnosis and management of peptic ulcer disease. *Clin Fam Pract*. 2004;6(3):569–587.

2.46. Peripheral Arterial Disease

Gey DC, Lesho EP, Manngold J. Management of peripheral arterial disease. *Am Fam Physician*. 2004;69(3):525–533.

Hiatt WR. Medical treatment of peripheral arterial disease and claudication. *N Engl J Med*. 2001;344(21):1608–1621.

2.47. Pneumonia (Community-acquired)

File TM. Community-acquired pneumonia. *Lancet*. 2003;362:1991–2001.

Green WK, Vande Waa JA. Bacterial pneumonia. In: Rakel RE, Bope ET, eds. *Conn's current therapy 2006*. Philadelphia: WB Saunders; 2006: 321–327.

Halm EA, Teirstein AS. Management of community-acquired pneumonia. *N Engl J Med*. 2002;347(25):2039–2045.

2.48. Sinusitis (Acute Bacterial)

Piccirillo JF. Acute bacterial sinusitis. *N Engl J Med*. 2004;351(9):902–910.

Scheid DC, Hamm RM. Acute bacterial rhinosinusitis in adults: Part I. Evaluation. *Am Fam Physician*. 2004;70(9):1685–1692.

Scheid DC, Hamm RM. Acute bacterial rhinosinusitis in adults: Part II. Treatment. *Am Fam Physician*. 2004;70(9):1697–1704, 1711–1712.

2.49. Skin Ailments—Acne Vulgaris

Feldman S, Careccia RE, Barham KL, et al. Diagnosis and treatment of acne. *Am Fam Physician*. 2004;69(9):2123–2130, 2135–2136.

2.50. Skin Ailments—Cellulitis

Stulberg DL, Penrod MA, Blatny RA. Common bacterial skin infections. *Am Fam Physician*. 2002;66(1):119–124.

Swartz MN. Cellulitis. *N Engl J Med*. 2004;350(9):904–912.

2.51. Skin Ailments—Dermatitis

Berger TG. Skin, hair, and nails. In Tierney LM, McPhee SJ, Papdakis MA, eds. *Current medical diagnosis and treatment*, 43rd ed. New York: Appleton & Lange/McGraw-Hill, 2004:81–144.

Correale CE, Walker C, Murphy L, et al. Atopic dermatitis: A review of diagnosis and treatment. *Am Fam Physician*. 1999;60(4):1191–1198, 1209–1210.

Ferri FF. Medication comparison tables. In: Ferri FF, ed. *Ferri: Practical guide to the care of the medical patient*, 6th ed. St. Louis: Mosby; 2004: 1119–1125.

Habif TP. Topical therapy and topical corticosteroids. In: Habif TP, ed. *Habif: Clinical dermatology*, 4th ed. Edinburgh: Mosby; 2004;23–40.

Johnson BA, Nunley JR. Treatment of seborrheic dermatitis. *Am Fam Physician*. 2000;61(9):2703–2710, 2713–2714.

Salim A, Eichenfield LF. Atopic dermatitis. In: Rakel RE, Bope ET, eds. *Conn's current therapy 2006*. Philadelphia: WB Saunders; 2006:1038–1041.

Sasseville D. Contact dermatitis. In: Rakel RE, Bope ET, eds. *Conn's current therapy 2006*. Philadelphia: WB Saunders; 2006:1052–1054.

2.52. Skin Ailments—Ectoparasites

Flinders DC, De Schweinitz P. Pediculosis and scabies. *Am Fam Physician*. 2004;69(2):341–350.

2.53. Skin Ailments—Pruritus

Yiannias JA, Conroy MP. Pruritus. In: Rakel RE, Bope ET, eds. *Conn's current therapy 2006*. Philadelphia: WB Saunders; 2006:39–42.

2.54. Skin Ailments—Tinea

Hebert AA. Fungal diseases of the skin. In: Rakel RE, Bope ET, eds. *Conn's current therapy 2006*. Philadelphia: WB Saunders; 2006:1021–1025.

Weinstein A, Berman B. Topical treatment of common superficial tinea infections. *Am Fam Physician*. 2002;65(10):2095–2102.

2.55. Stye (Hordeolum)

Masci JR. Hordeolum (Stye). In: Ferri FF, ed. *Ferri: Ferri's clinical advisor: Instant diagnosis and treatment*, 8th ed. Philadelphia: Mosby; 2006: 399.

2.56. Urinary Incontinence

Culligan PJ, Heit M. Urinary incontinence in women: Evaluation and management. *Am Fam Physician*. 2000;62(11):2433–2444, 2452.

Fantl JA, Newman DK, Colling J, et al. *Urinary Incontinence in Adults: Acute and Chronic Management*. Clinical Practice Guideline, No. 2, 1996 Update, AHCPR Publication No. 96-0682, Public Health Service, Agency for Health Care Policy and Research, Rockville, MD.

Galloway NTM. Urinary Incontinence. In: Rakel RE, Bope ET, eds. *Conn's current therapy 2006*. Philadelphia: WB Saunders; 2006:841–847.

Gerber GS, Brendler CB. Evaluation of the urologic patient: History, physical examination, and urinalysis. In Walsh PC, ed. *Campbell's urology*, 8th ed. Philadelphia: WB Saunders; 2002:83–110.

Rakel D. Benign prostatic hyperplasia. In: Rakel D, ed. *Rakel: Integrative medicine*, 1st ed. Philadelphia: WB Saunders; 2003:393–397.

2.57. Urinary Tract Infection

Norrby R. Urinary Tract Infections. In: Goldman L, Ausiello D, eds. *Cecil textbook of medicine*, 22nd ed. Philadelphia: WB Saunders; 2004:1909–1913.

Orenstein R, Wong ES. Urinary tract infections in adults. *Am Fam Physician*. 1999;59(5):1225–1234, 1237.

2.58. Vaginitis

Corigliano MA. Gonorrhea. In: Ferri FF, ed. *Ferri: Ferri's clinical advisor: Instant diagnosis and treatment*, 8th ed. Philadelphia: Mosby; 2006:348.

Schmid GP. Gonorrhea. In: Rakel RE, Bope ET, eds. *Conn's current therapy 2006*. Philadelphia: WB Saunders; 2006:906–908.

Sobel JD. Vaginitis. *N Engl J Med*. 1997;337(26):1896–1903.

2.59. Wound Care

Beckrich K, Aronovitch SA. Hospital-acquired pressure ulcers: A comparison of costs in medical *vs.* surgical patients. *Nurs Econ*. 1999;17(5):263–271.

Brook I. Management of human and animal bite wounds: An overview. *Adv Skin Wound Care*. 2005;18(4):197–203.

Lammers RL. Principles of Wound Management. In Roberts JR, Hedges JR, eds. *Clinical procedures in emergency medicine*, 4th ed. Philadelphia: WB Saunders; 2004:623–654.

Niezgoda JA, Mendez-Eastman S. The effective management of pressure ulcers. *Adv Skin Wound Care*. 2006;19(Suppl 1):3–15.

Presutti RJ. Prevention and treatment of dog bites. *Am Fam Physician*. 2001;63(8):1567–1574.

Swartz MN. Cellulitis. *N Engl J Med*. 2004;350(9):904–912.

Thomas, DR. Pressure ulcers. In: Rakel RE. Bope ET, eds. *Conn's current therapy 2006*. Philadelphia: WB Saunders; 2006:1036–1038.

SECTION 3

3.1. Syndrome of Inappropriate Secretion of Antidiuretic Hormone

Delva NJ, Crammer JL. Polydipsia in chronic psychiatric patients. *Br J Psychiatry Suppl*. 1988;152:242–245.

Fukagawa M, Kurokawa K, Papdakis K. Fluid and electrolyte disorders. In McPhee SJ, Papadakis MA, Tierney LM Jr, eds. *Current medical diagnosis and treatment*, New York: Appleton & Lange, McGraw-Hill, 2007:887–917.

Jawetz R. Water, water everywhere… The etiology and treatment of polydipsia and hyponatremia. *P & S Medical Review*. 1999;6:1.

Vieweg WVR. Treatment strategies in the polydipsia-hyponatremia syndrome. *J Clin Psychiatry*. 1994;55:154–160.

3.2. Neuroleptic Malignant Syndrome

Gurrera RJ. Sympathoadrenal hyperactivity and the etiology of neuroleptic malignant syndrome. *Am J Psychiatry*. 1999;156(2):169–180.Feb;

Tonkonogy J, Sholevar D. *Neuroleptic Malignant Syndrome.* Emedicine on-line. May 2006.

3.3. Serotonin Syndrome

Boyer EW, Shannon M. Current concepts: The serotonin syndrome. *N Engl J Med.* 2005;352(11):1112–1120.

3.4. Noradrenergic Syndrome of Early Tricyclic Syndrome

Fitzgerald M. SSRI discontinuation syndrome. *J Inform Pharmacother.* 2001;7:303–304.

Haddad, PM. *The SSRI Discontinuation Syndrome: Literature Review and Provisional Diagnostic Criteria.* Presented at: XXIst Collegium Internationale Neuro-Psychopharmacologicum Congress. July 12–16, 1998; Glasgow, Scotland. Reprinted in *International Drug Therapy Newsletter.* 1998;33:46.

Judge R, Parry MG, Quail D, et al. Discontinuation symptoms: Comparison of brief interruption in fluoxetine and paroxetine treatment. *Int Clin Psychopharmacol.* 2002;17(5):217–225.

Schatzberg AF, Haddad P, Kaplan EM, et al. Serotonin reuptake inhibitor discontinuation syndrome: A hypothetical definition. *J Clin Psychiatry.* 1997;58(Suppl 7):5–10.

3.5. Selective Serotonin Reuptake Inhibitors Withdrawal Syndrome

Fitzgerald M. SSRI discontinuation syndrome. *J Inform Pharmacother.* 2001;7:303–304.

Haddad, PM. *The SSRI Discontinuation Syndrome: Literature Review and Provisional Diagnostic Criteria.* Presented at: XXIst Collegium Internationale Neuro-Psychopharmacologicum Congress. July 12–16, 1998; Glasgow, Scotland. Reprinted in *International Drug Therapy Newsletter.* 1998;33:46.

Judge R, Parry MG, Quail D, et al. Discontinuation symptoms: Comparison of brief interruption in fluoxetine and paroxetine treatment. *Int Clin Psychopharmacol.* 2002;17(5):217–225.

Schatzberg AF, Haddad P, Kaplan EM, et al. Serotonin reuptake inhibitor discontinuation syndrome: A hypothetical definition. *J Clin Psychiatry.* 1997;58(Suppl 7):5–10.

3.6. Heatstroke

Barrow MW, Clark KA. Heat-related illnesses. *Am Fam Physician.* 1998; 58(3):749–756, 759.

Bouchama A, Knochel JP. Medical progress: Heatstroke. *N Engl J Med.* 2002;346:1978–1988.

Epstein Y, Albukrek D, Kalmovitc B, et al. Heat intolerance induced by antidepressants. *Ann N Y Acad Sci.* 1997;813:553–558.

Helman RS, Habal R. *Heatstroke.* Emedicine online, Jun 2005.

3.7. Heat Exhaustion

Barrow MW, Clark KA. Heat-Related Illnesses. *Am Fam Physician.* 1998; 58(3):749–756, 759. Sept.

3.8. Lithium-Induced Neurotoxic "Syndrome"

Adityanjee, Munshi KR, Thampy A. The syndrome of irreversible lithium-effectuated neurotoxicity. *Clin Neuropharmacol.* 2005:28(1):38–49.

Broussolle E, Seitey A, Moene Y, et al. Reversible Creutzfelt Jacob like syndrome induced by lithium and levodopa treatment. *J Neurol Neurosurg Psychiatry.* 1989;52:686–687.

Cookson J. Use of antipsychotic drugs and lithium in mania. *Br J Psychiatry Suppl.* 2001;178:148–156.

Linakis JG. *Lithium Toxicity.* Emedicine online, June 2006.

Okusa MD, Crystal LJ. Clinical manifestations and management of acute lithium intoxication. *American Journal of Medicine,* 1994;97(4):383–389.

Smith SJM, Kocen RS. A Creutzfelt Jakob like syndrome due to lithium toxicity. *J Neurol Neurosurg Psychiatry.* 1988;51:120–123.

Appendix I: Monitoring for Psychiatric Medications

Bauer Mark S. *Field guide to psychiatric assessment and treatment.* Philadelphia: Lippincott Williams & Wilkins; 2003:262–334.

Nasrallah HA, Newcomer JW. Atypical antipsychotics and metabolic dysregulation: Evaluating the risk/benefit equation and improving the standard of care. *J Clin Psychopharmacol.* 2004;24(Suppl 5):S7–S14.

Rosenbaum JF, Arana GW, Hyman SE, et al. *Handbook of psychiatric drug therapy,* 5th ed. Philadelphia: Lippincott Williams & Wilkins; 2005; 37.

Sadock BJ, Sadock VA. Chapter 7.4. Laboratory tests in psychiatry. In: Sadock BJ, Sadock VA, eds. *Kaplan and sadock's synopsis of psychiatry,* 9th ed. Philadelphia: Lippincott Williams & Wilkins; 2003:260–274.

INDEX